Psychiatric Services in
Correctional
Facilities

THIRD EDITION

The American Psychiatric Association Work Group to Revise the APA Guidelines on Psychiatric Services in Correctional Facilities

Robert L. Trestman, Ph.D., M.D., *Chair*
Michael K. Champion, M.D.
Elizabeth Ford, M.D.
Jeffrey L. Metzner, M.D.
Cassandra F. Newkirk, M.D., M.B.A.
Joseph V. Penn, M.D.
Debra A. Pinals, M.D.
Charles Scott, M.D.
Roberta E. Stellman, M.D.
Henry C. Weinstein, M.D.
Robert Weinstock, M.D.
Kenneth L. Appelbaum, M.D., *Consultant*
John L. Young, M.D., M.Th., *Consultant*

Psychiatric Services in
Correctional Facilities

THIRD EDITION

American Psychiatric Association

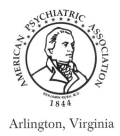

Arlington, Virginia

Copyright © 2016 American Psychiatric Association

ALL RIGHTS RESERVED

Manufactured in the United States of America on acid-free paper

19 18 17 16 15   5 4 3 2 1

First Edition

Typeset in Adobe's Baskerville BE and HelveticaNeuLT Std

American Psychiatric Publishing
A Division of American Psychiatric Association
1000 Wilson Boulevard
Arlington, VA 22209-3901
www.appi.org

Library of Congress Cataloging-in-Publication Data

American Psychiatric Association. Work Group to Revise the APA Guidelines on Psychiatric Services in Correctional Facilities, author.

Psychiatric services in correctional facilities / The American Psychiatric Association Work Group to Revise the APA Guidelines on Psychiatric Services in Correctional Facilities. – Third edition.

p. ; cm.

Preceded by Psychiatric services in jails and prisons : a task force report of the American Psychiatric Association / American Psychiatric Association, Task Force to Revise the APA Guidelines on Psychiatric Services in jails and Prisons. c2000.

Includes bibliographical references and index.

ISBN 978-0-89042-464-3 (pbk. : alk. paper)

I. American Psychiatric Association. Task Force to Revise the APA Guidelines on Psychiatric Services in Jails and Prisons. Psychiatric services in jails and prisons. Preceded by (work): II. Title.

[DNLM: 1. Mental Health Services–organization & administration–United States. 2. Delivery of Health Care–organization & administration–United States. 3. Practice Guidelines as Topic–United States. 4. Prisons–United States. 5. Psychotherapy–organization & administration–United States. WM 30 AA1]

RC451.4.P68

365'.66–dc23

2015016058

British Library Cataloguing in Publication Data

A CIP record is available from the British Library.

Contents

CONTRIBUTORS

Kenneth L. Appelbaum, M.D.
Clinical Professor of Psychiatry; Director, Correctional Mental Health Policy and Research, Center for Health Policy and Research, Commonwealth Medicine; University of Massachusetts Medical School, Shrewsbury, Massachusetts

Michael K. Champion, M.D.
Forensic Chief, Hawai'i Department of Health, Adult Mental Health Division; Associate Clinical Professor of Psychiatry, John A. Burns School of Medicine, University of Hawai'i at Manoa, Honolulu, Hawaii

Elizabeth Ford, M.D.
Executive Director of Mental Health, Correctional Health Services, New York City Department of Health and Mental Hygiene; Clinical Associate Professor, New York University School of Medicine, New York, New York

Jeffrey L. Metzner, M.D.
Clinical Professor of Psychiatry, Department of Psychiatry, University of Colorado School of Medicine, Denver, Colorado

Cassandra F. Newkirk, M.D., M.B.A., DFAPA
Chief Clinical Officer, Correct Care LLC, Deerfield Beach, Florida

Joseph V. Penn, M.D., CCHP, FAPA
Director, Mental Health Services, UTMB Correctional Managed Care; Clinical Professor of Psychiatry, Department of Psychiatry, University of Texas Medical Branch, Galveston, Texas

Debra A. Pinals, M.D.
Assistant Commissioner of Forensic Services, Massachusetts Department of Mental Health; Associate Professor of Psychiatry, University of Massachusetts Medical School, Worcester, Massachusetts

Charles Scott, M.D.
Professor of Clinical Psychiatry and Chief, Division of Psychiatry and the Law, Department of Psychiatry and Behavioral Sciences, University of California, Davis

Roberta E. Stellman, M.D.

Robert L. Trestman, Ph.D., M.D., FAPA
Professor of Medicine, Psychiatry, and Nursing, and Executive Director, Correctional Managed Health Care, University of Connecticut, UCONN Health, Farmington, Connecticut

Henry C. Weinstein, M.D.
Clinical Professor of Psychiatry and Director, Program in Psychiatry and the Law, Department of Psychiatry, New York University Medical Center, New York, New York

Robert Weinstock, M.D.
Clinical Professor, Department of Psychiatry and Biobehavioral Science, University of California, Los Angeles, Los Angeles, California

John L. Young, M.D., M.Th.
Clinical Professor of Psychiatry, Department of Psychiatry, Yale University School of Medicine, New Haven, Connecticut

Disclosure of Competing Interests

Jeffrey L. Metzner, M.D., consults to various state department of corrections regarding their mental health services, as well as plaintiffs and defendants in litigation involving correctional mental health issues. Dr. Metzner also monitors various correctional mental health systems for federal courts on implementation of court-ordered mental health services.

Robert Weinstock, M.D., is immediate past president of the American Academy of Psychiatry and the Law.

The following contributors to this book have indicated no competing interests to disclose during the year preceding manuscript submission:
Kenneth L. Appelbaum, M.D.
Michael K. Champion, M.D.
Elizabeth Ford, M.D.
Cassandra F. Newkirk, M.D., M.B.A., DFAPA
Joseph V. Penn, M.D., CCHP, FAPA
Debra A. Pinals, M.D.
Charles Scott, M.D.
Roberta E. Stellman, M.D.
Robert L. Trestman, Ph.D., M.D., FAPA
John L. Young, M.D., M.Th.

PREFACE

This document was a long time in the making. In the 15 years since the last edition, there has been an evolution in correctional mental health care, continued and increasing rates of incarceration of individuals with mental illness, ongoing criminalization of substance use disorders, and a lack of accessible and appropriate care in the community. The contributors to this document spent many hours reviewing the issues, challenges, and concerns of correctional psychiatrists in this evolving field. We have worked to get input from multiple sources and perspectives. Given the challenging nature and scope of this endeavor, it may be surprising that so much of the content was reached with consensus support. I believe it also reflects the fact that the field itself is maturing.

Several items bear noting here. The first is the obvious change in the title from the second edition: no longer limited explicitly to just jails and prisons, the title now incorporates lockups and adult detention centers into the more global term "correctional facilities." This change reflects the Work Group's belief that the guidelines herein apply appropriately to all of these adult incarceration settings.

All of the sections were reviewed and were extensively rewritten to reflect changes and current status. Many new sections were added to address evolving challenges and concerns. These sections include clinical issues such as nonsuicidal self-injury, infectious disease, sleep disorders, and attention-deficit/hyperactivity disorder. Clinically significant populations that are now specifically addressed include lesbian, gay, bisexual, and transgender (LGBT) persons; veterans; and individuals with intellectual or developmental disabilities. New management and programmatic topics include hospice, mental illness and segregation, seclusion and restraint, telepsychiatry, and spiritual lives of inmates.

These guidelines are just that: guidelines. This document is not a set of standards, policies, or procedures. It is intended to serve and support psychiatrists working in correctional settings as they grapple with the many opportunities to care for very disadvantaged populations in environments where the primary focus is safety and security. We hope it provides a useful resource to the many dedicated and talented psychiatrists providing care and shaping the mental health services in the thousands of correctional settings throughout the United States.

Robert L. Trestman, Ph.D., M.D., FAPA

INTRODUCTION

Overview

When the first edition of these guidelines was published in September 1989, an editorial in *The American Journal of Psychiatry* noted, "On any day, our nation's jails and prisons hold an estimated 1.2 million men and women." In 2012, this number had almost doubled to 2.2 million. Contributing factors to this substantial increase included harsher sanctions associated with the "war on drugs" and the general public's attitude toward "getting tough on crime." In addition, more rigid sentencing policies had removed judicial discretion regarding sentence lengths and limited parole board discretion in the release of inmates.

Many studies have consistently demonstrated that about 16% of inmates in jails and prisons have serious mental illnesses and are in need of psychiatric care (Diamond et al. 2001; Ditton 1999; Fazel and Danesh 2002; Steadman et al. 2009; Trestman et al. 2007). Upward of 700,000 men and women entering the U.S. criminal justice system each year have active symptoms of serious mental disorders, and studies have suggested that up to 3% (approximately 66,000) are actively psychotic. Approximately three of every four incarcerated persons with a serious mental illness have a co-occurring substance use disorder (e.g., Baillargeon et al. 2010). Inmates with mental illness are likely to stay incarcerated longer, and return to prison more rapidly, than persons without mental disorders (Cloyes et al. 2010). What are our duties and responsibilities as psychiatrists to address this situation? How do we live up to our personal moral principles, our professional ethics, and our public service obligations in the face of these overwhelming numbers? These questions drove the creation of this document as the American Psychiatric Association (APA) seeks to provide leadership in addressing the needs of this often disenfranchised group and guidance to psychiatric and mental health professionals working in correctional settings.

The vast majority of psychiatrists who practice in jails and prisons function almost exclusively as diagnosticians and prescribers, yet a need and an important opportunity exist for psychiatrists to expand their roles. As a profession, we must address the relationship between mental illness and incarceration. Given our extensive training and broad skill set, psychiatrists may benefit systems by assuming greater leadership positions. As physician leaders, managers, and directors, psychiatrists can more effectively advocate for their patients and help to shape optimal care delivery systems that empower patients and support successful transition back to the community.

This document is intended to encourage action and to provide comprehensive guidance on how to fulfill these responsibilities to ourselves, our profession, and these often underserved patients. We have new technology for treatment and care coordination. We have the knowledge base and the skill set to effectively intervene. Yet limited resources and public and professional resistance often impede an appropriate response. We hope that this document will help mobilize additional resources and encourage the informed action that overcomes resistance to enhanced care. We feel inspired by the high quality and humane services delivered by our dedicated colleagues across the United States, and we believe that even greater involvement by our profession can make an enormous difference.

Clarification of Terms

Correctional Facilities

For the purposes of these guidelines, *correctional facilities* include

- Lockups
- Jails
- State and federal prisons
- U.S. Immigration and Customs Enforcement (ICE) detention centers
- Bureau of Indian Affairs detention centers
- U.S. military prisons, jails, and detention centers

When a psychiatrist treats individuals, regardless of setting, they become patients. All ethical obligations to patients therefore hold. Individuals in correctional settings are generally referred to as *detainees* (pretrial) or *offenders* (postsentencing). For ease of discussion, this text uses the term inmates to refer to both populations. The terms psychiatric, mental health, and behavioral health are commonly used to describe clinical services provided to persons with psychiatric conditions in correctional facilities. These guidelines define the term psychiatric services in correctional facilities as all mental health services, including substance use services, provided in correctional facilities, with emphasis on the unique role of psychiatrists in the delivery of these services.

Jails, Lockups, and Detention Centers

A *jail* generally is defined as a facility where an individual is confined either while awaiting trial or, in most jurisdictions, while serving a sentence of 1 year or less. These facilities are usually under the jurisdiction of the county or municipality in which they are located. Jails, lockups, and detention centers are high-volume facilities. There are about 3,350 jails around the country, processing approximately 10 million people each year. Jails differ greatly in size, ranging from facilities holding fewer than 50 inmates to complexes capable of holding more than 10,000. *Lockups* are typically small, short-term holding areas in a police station for individuals awaiting arraignment in a court. *Detention centers* are here broadly defined as institutions where people are held for (generally) short periods, in particular illegal immigrants or refugees. Confinement in a jail, lockup, or detention center may occur for different reasons. For example, some jurisdictions use jails to house people for civil charges, public health reasons, detention for ICE, or as temporary housing for state and federal inmates. Each purpose can result in differing periods and conditions of confinement.

Confinement in a jail, lockup, or detention center usually takes place shortly after arrest, and the stress level and health needs of detainees may be extremely high. Furthermore, conditions that may have been present at the time of the arrest, such as intoxication or psychosis, are likely to still be acute. These factors increase the risk of suicidal behavior, violence, and death—often related to intoxication with drugs or alcohol. Individuals with acute mental health needs require an immediate response. In addition, inmates may experience mental health problems or psychiatric crises during their incarcerations. Issues may arise concerning treatment, restraint and seclusion, safety of the staff and detainees, or emergency medical and psychiatric needs of inmates. Psychiatrists may need to file court petitions for involuntary treatment with medication or involuntary hospitalization on release from these facilities.

In jails, lockups, and detention centers, the core components of essential psychiatric services are screening, referral, assessment, evaluation, treatment, and community reentry planning. Communities throughout the United States are seeing a decrease in the number of inpatient psychiatric hospital beds and an increasing number of acutely mentally ill persons in these settings. Community hospitals frequently refuse to accept violent or aggressive inmates, forcing jails, lockups, and detention centers to provide more complicated services to meet the needs of these inmates.

Prisons

A *prison* is generally defined as a correctional facility where an individual is confined to serve a sentence, usually in excess of 1 year. In contrast to jails, which are usually under the jurisdiction of the county or municipality in which they are located, most prisons are operated by state governments. The federal government also operates its own prison system, the Federal Bureau of Prisons. There are many fewer prisons than jails, and prisons usually house many inmates (often more than 1,000).

In contrast to inmates in jails, lockups, and detention centers, prison inmates often have been in the criminal justice system for an extended period. By the time inmates arrive at prison, they often have spent a long time in custody and have different mental health issues from recently arrested inmates. For example, they may have a lower incidence of acute psychotic states and better psychological adaptation to the loss of liberty, but they may have more stress due to recent sentencing, facility transfer, or greater geographic separation from family and friends. The prevalence of long-term psychotic illnesses in prison, however, is comparable to that in other correctional facilities, and prison inmates recently apprehended for parole violations have mental health issues commonly seen in other facilities. The components of essential mental health services in prisons are the same as in other correctional facilities: screening, assessment, referral, evaluation, treatment, and community reentry planning.

Serious Mental Illness

Health care organizations (e.g., the Society of Correctional Physicians, the National Institute of Mental Health, the National Commission on Correctional Health Care, Substance Abuse and Mental Health Services Administration) define *serious mental illness* (SMI) in different ways, on the basis of distinct perspectives and purposes. Although these differences are a natural reflection of an evolving field, they contribute to challenges in developing consensus positions necessary to advance and standardize correctional mental health care practice. Establishing a consistent definition of SMI in the correctional context is important for epidemiological purposes, needs assessment, and mental health system planning.

Psychiatric disorders that include psychotic symptoms, at least on an intermittent basis, are uniformly considered to meet criteria for SMI. Schizophrenia, schizoaffective disorder, and delusional disorder are examples of such serious mental illnesses. Other mental or emotional disorders (e.g., major depression, bipolar disorder, posttraumatic stress disorder), whether acute or chronic, that result in serious distress or serious functional impairment that substantially interferes with or limits one or more major life activities almost always meet criteria for SMI. Some prisoners with severe personality disorders, cognitive disorders, or adjustment disorders will meet such criteria either temporarily or chronically.

Clinical judgment must always be employed in determining the appropriate care for individuals, whether or not they meet SMI criteria.

A Road Map

This third edition of the APA's *Psychiatric Services in Correctional Facilities* has three parts. The first part, "Principles Governing the Delivery of Psychiatric Services in Correctional Facilities," discusses foundational principles that apply to providing care in all correctional facilities. The second part, "Guidelines for Psychiatric Services in Correctional Facilities," outlines three basic types of services that should be provided: 1) screening, referral, and evaluation; 2) treatment; and 3) community reentry planning. The third part, "Special Applications of the Principles and Guidelines," applies the principles and guidelines established in the first two parts to specific disorders/syndromes, patient populations, housing locations, treatment modalities, and special needs of inmates.

PART 1

Principles Governing the Delivery of Psychiatric Services in Correctional Facilities

Introduction

The principles outlined here are intended as a foundational framework to guide the delivery of psychiatric services in correctional facilities. These principles are necessary elements of constitutionally acceptable provision of care. They serve only as compass points for psychiatrists navigating the complex landscape of correctional mental health care. They are not intended to serve as operational standards.

The Legal Context

A basic understanding of the legal context of psychiatric services in correctional facilities helps frame the principles and guidelines that follow. This context is unique: in no other setting is treatment constitutionally required. The following discussion provides a brief overview of legal decisions that drive the provision of clinical services in correctional settings. A more extensive treatment of this subject is available elsewhere (e.g., Cohen 2011).

Right to Treatment

Incarcerated persons have a constitutionally derived right to treatment for their serious medical needs, which include serious mental illness (SMI). Whenever a county, state, or federal governmental entity takes custody of a person, it has a duty to provide for the necessities of life that the person otherwise is unable to obtain. Such necessities include food, clothing, shelter, and medical care. Failure to provide medical care in this context has been interpreted as cruel and unusual punishment. The U.S. Supreme Court has recognized that pretrial detainees have a due process right to not be punished and that convicted inmates have a right to not be punished in a cruel and unusual manner. Courts have interpreted the due process clause of the 14th Amendment as the constitutional standard regarding the right to treatment of pretrial detainees. The 8th Amendment of the U.S. Constitution prohibiting cruel and unusual punishment serves as the basis for a prisoner's right to treatment. In the landmark case *Estelle v. Gamble* (429 U.S. 97 [1976]), the U.S. Supreme Court held that it is unconstitutional for prison officials to be deliberately indifferent to the serious medical needs of individuals in their custody. Subsequent decisions established the dimensions of this constitutional right and the government's duty to provide it. *Bowring v. Godwin* (551 F.2d 44 [4th Cir. 1977]) was the first federal court decision to extend this requirement to psychiatric care by equating mental health care with medical treatment. Since then, numerous federal and state court decisions have equated medical and psychiatric care, although the Supreme Court has yet to specifically address this issue. In *Farmer v. Brennan* (511 U.S. 825 [1994]) the Court later defined the federal standard as *deliberate indifference:* a knowing disregard of an excessive risk to an inmate's health or safety.

A common method for addressing asserted violations of inmates' rights is the federal civil rights statute 42 U.S.C. § 1983 with claims filed in federal court. Physicians can be sued for violating the constitutional rights of inmates under Section 1983. For the psychiatrist practicing in a correctional setting, it is important to know that beyond providing for inmates' constitutional rights, physicians have an additional duty to practice within the standard of care for their profession. Negligence in failing to provide services within the standard of care may not support a constitutional claim but may be pursued as a malpractice claim based on state law and filed in state court.

Adequate Care

Federal decisions that establish the framework and specific criteria for constitutionally adequate psychiatric care in jails and prisons within their geographic jurisdictions include the U.S. Supreme Court case *Ruiz v. Estelle* (503 F. Supp. 1265 [S.D. Tex. 1980]), a class action suit that established six essential elements of minimally adequate mental health services:

- Systematic screening and evaluation
- Treatment that is more than mere seclusion or close supervision

- Participation by trained mental health professionals
- An accurate, complete, and confidential record
- Safeguards against psychotropic medications that are prescribed in dangerous amounts, without adequate supervision, or in an otherwise inappropriate manner
- A suicide prevention program

In *Langley v. Coughlin* (888 F. 2d 252 [1989]; 709 F. Supp. 482 [1989]; 715 F. Supp. 522 [1989]), the Court established specific criteria that, if not met, could provide a basis for successful inmate legal claims. Many of these criteria explicitly require providing for secondary or supportive rights that are necessary to facilitate the primary right to a diagnosis and treatment. Examples include taking a psychiatric history, maintaining a medical record, diagnosing mental conditions properly, and placing inmates experiencing a mental health crisis in an observation setting. *Langley* also explicitly requires that treatment not be limited to psychotropic medication.

Madrid v. Gomez (889 F.Supp. 1146 [1995]) added several factors that may determine the constitutionality of a correctional mental health system:

- Inmates must have a means of making their needs known to the medical staff.
- There must be sufficient staffing to allow individualized treatment of each inmate with SMI.
- An inmate must have speedy access to services.
- There must be a system of quality assurance.
- Staff must be competent and well trained.
- There must be a system of responding to emergencies and preventing suicides.

Many correctional systems have developed quality improvement programs, related to both court orders and good practice, which are expected to incorporate a quality assurance component.

Treatment Over Objection

The U.S. Supreme Court in *Washington v. Harper* (494 U.S. 210 [1990]) recognized a constitutionally permissible model under which an inmate in a prison may be administered treatment over objection. The Court held that an appropriate internal administrative hearing rather than a judicial review satisfies due process requirements. This decision led to the development of so-called *Harper* hearings that provide a review by an independent committee, with procedural safeguards including a right to notice, an opportunity for the prisoner to present evidence and cross-examine witnesses, a right to have the assistance of an advisor, and a right to appeal. *Harper* does not require a lack of decisional competence or consideration of less intrusive means of intervention. In jurisdictions that do not require transfer to a psychiatric hospital to initiate treatment over objection, some jail systems have also adopted a *Harper* process for treatment over objection.

The substantive and procedural approach found permissible in *Harper*, however, fails to meet legal standards in all jurisdictions. For example, some states require lack of decisional competence and a judicial determination of best interest or substituted judgment before any individual, including inmates, can receive involuntary psychotropic medications in nonemergency situations. Correctional psychiatrists need to be familiar with the legal standards where they practice.

Conditions of Confinement

Rates of incarceration have escalated over the past several decades, straining the ability to house the numbers of individuals placed in correctional systems. Overcrowding is commonplace and contributes to barriers to accessing care and basic services. The psychological and emotional impact of resulting conditions of confinement has received increasing attention. In *Brown v. Plata* (131 S. Ct. 1910 [2011]), the U.S. Supreme Court found that overcrowding was a significant contributing factor in creating barriers to delivering adequate health care in the California Department of Corrections and Rehabilitation. The Court held that a mandated population cap was necessary to address the violation of inmates' rights.

In addition to constitutional mandates, other legal requirements apply to mental health services in correctional facilities. These include federal statutes such as the Americans with Disabilities Act and state requirements established through state constitutions, statutes, and regulations. Furthermore, the Civil Rights of Institutionalized Persons Act provides an avenue for the U.S. Department of Justice to investigate alleged violations in state institutions.

Access to Mental Health Care and Treatment

Timely and effective access to screening, evaluation, and mental health treatment is the hallmark of adequate mental health care. The first edition of these guidelines emphasized this fundamental principle of adequate mental health care in correctional facilities. Investments in clinical resources and programming will have little impact if barriers to assessment, diagnosis, and follow-up care exist. Adequate and appropriate access to mental health treatment means that patients have no unreasonable barriers to receiving services. Examples of unreasonable barriers include disincentives, including fees that deter a patient from seeking care for legitimate mental health needs; interference with the prompt transmittal of a patient's oral or written request for care; unreasonable delays before patients are seen by mental health staff or outside consultants; insufficient custody staff to transport inmates to clinic; inadequate waiting room space; and punishment for seeking or refusing care.

Clinical autonomy is another key element of appropriate access to mental health care. Clinical autonomy occurs when clinical decisions and actions regarding mental health care provided to inmates are the sole responsibility of qualified mental health professionals (QMHPs). A QMHP is someone privileged for independent assessment on the basis of discipline-specific professional standards and state statutes.

Every correctional system should have a mechanism for monitoring access to psychiatric care. Efforts to improve access include routine orientation and training for custody staff on common manifestations of mental illness and for inmates on how to use the institutional health care system. Encouraging and supporting a collaborative relationship and good communication between mental health and custody staff will maximize the likelihood of delivering quality clinical services. Mental health clinicians, nursing and other health care staff, and custody personnel are partners in providing safe and effective services to inmates. It is essential that they align their efforts to identify inmates with mental illness and coordinate an effective response.

Quality of Care

The fundamental policy goal for correctional mental health care is to provide the same quality of mental health services to each patient in the criminal justice system that *should be available* in the community. This policy goal is deliberately higher than the "community standard" that is called for in various legal contexts, because resource restrictions on community care can sometimes limit the adequacy of available services. Correctional systems provide additional challenges not present in the community, given that incarcerated persons have no options for care other than what is provided in the correctional facility.

Quality Assessment and Performance Improvement

It is imperative that facility staff gather and assess information about the prevalence and incidence of mental illness, including demographic and clinical characteristics associated with such illness. This information is critical for needs assessments, program administration, and advocacy within and outside of the correctional setting.

Each facility or administrative authority should prepare a regularly updated quality improvement plan that systematically sets out to review and improve the quality of mental health services. The efficiency and effectiveness of the use of staff and resources in service delivery are key elements in such a plan. Quality assurance and improvement activities include credentialing, review of service access and use, documentation and review of records, resource management, morbidity and mortality review, continuing education opportunities, identification and prevention of risk, and monitoring and review of high-risk critical procedures such as overriding treatment refusals and responding to emergencies. It is recommended that psychiatrists involved in direct patient care, supervision, and management be involved in the creation of the quality improvement plan. Only psychiatrists have the depth and breadth of training to assess fully the needs of inmates with mental illness.

Facilities are encouraged to participate in relevant accreditation programs that provide guidance and quality-of-care oversight. There are several national accreditation programs, including the National Commission on Correctional Health Care (NCCHC) and the Joint Commission, along with state-specific and local accrediting agencies. Although such accreditation does not guarantee adequate mental health services or compliance with recommended guidelines, regular monitoring represents an effort to enhance the quality of care.

Prioritizing Resources

Many factors determine allocation of correctional mental health treatment resources, including resource availability, facility size, service organization, facility mission, inmate length of stay, and governing legal action or court oversight.

The highest priority for care should be patients with SMIs, whose symptoms lead to dangerous, self-harming, or other problematic behavior and who may require triage to a higher level of care. However, these individuals typically represent a minority of patients. Inmates who do not have SMI or who are not behaving in a manner that places others, themselves, or the institution at risk may still experience profound suffering and should receive appropriate resources and treatment planning.

There is a frequent tension between security and treatment in correctional settings. Facility administrators and clinicians should attempt to make the best use of resources to deliver priority care without unduly compromising safety or security.

Staffing

Adequate numbers of appropriately trained mental health professionals, performing duties for which they are trained and authorized, must be present in every correctional facility. Staffing must be adequate to ensure that every inmate with SMI or in psychiatric or emotional crisis has timely access to evaluation by a competent mental health professional. Psychiatrists must play an integral leadership role in the development, implementation, delivery, and quality oversight of this care.

Psychiatrists are a critical and necessary component of any correctional mental health delivery system. Diagnostic evaluation and prescription of psychotropic medications are frequently the most significant mental health treatment interventions for inmates with SMI. Psychotropic medications can be prescribed and monitored most effectively and safely by psychiatrists, who are trained in the medical evaluation and management of mental illness and comorbidities. In addition, psychiatrists are uniquely trained to assess and address the biopsychosocial needs of inmates with mental illness, who frequently have disturbances in all three of these dimensions. This is particularly important given the high rates of SMI and acute and chronic medical conditions in correctional facilities. Psychiatrists receive considerable foundational and continuing education in providing care that meets the best interests of their patients, in navigating the complex landscape of confidentiality, and in maintaining professional integrity in challenging health care environments. Psychiatrists are held to high ethical standards (American Psychiatric Association 2013b) and frequently assume leadership roles.

Psychiatry staffing levels in correctional facilities are complicated algorithms that vary on the basis of clinical acuity and patient needs, system organization, physical plants, acuity of care delivery, resource availability, and population characteristics. The factors that have impacts on psychiatric staffing in correctional settings are facility specific. These factors include type of facility (jail, intake facility, prison), size of facility (e.g., average daily population [ADP] less than 50, ADP greater than 1,000), inmate turnover rate, location of facility, program space availability, security level of facility (higher security demands restrict movement and may significantly reduce clinician productivity), and care delivery model (e.g., team vs. individual practitioner). Specifically, a few of the many factors that may reduce psychiatric productivity through reduced access to patients include the need to individually cuff, shackle, and escort some inmates by custody personnel; the need to have limited numbers of inmates in any waiting area; the wait for count and other locked-down time periods; and the wait for multiple doors along the path from cell to examination room to be unlocked by central control staff. Higher-security facilities and high-risk patient populations pose additional safety-related challenges in staff recruitment, retention, and productivity. Small, medium-security prisons with stable populations allow for greater productivity.

There are no prevailing national standards for psychiatric staffing in correctional or other settings. Nevertheless, courts and regulatory agencies, court monitors, and health consultants frequently seek to establish staffing ratios in correctional settings in order to comply with constitutionally mandated minimally acceptable medical care. Governmental agencies with oversight of correctional settings often seek such ratios to assess their budgetary needs. Correctional facilities have historically not had enough psychiatrists to adequately provide the services described here.

In practice, a facility-specific staffing needs analysis is a fundamental step in determining the actual psychiatric staffing required to meet the standards of care in any given facility.

Correctional administrators and other leaders need guidance about adequate psychiatric staffing. Needs and type vary on the basis of patient acuity and treatment need, patient volume and turnover, facility location (whether services will be provided on site, via telepsychiatry, or a combination of both modalities), the role and function of the facility, the targeted inmate population, any unique or specialized unit or facility treatment/rehabilitative mission, and changes to any of the above. Although it is very difficult to establish exact psychiatrist-to-patient ratios, the amount of psychiatric time must be sufficient to ensure that there is no unreasonable delay in patients receiving necessary care, and all relevant and necessary psychiatric functions must be met. On the basis of 15 years of experience in the field since the publication of the second edition of *Psychiatric Services in Jails and Prisons,* the following are recommended basic guidelines regarding psychiatric staffing requirements.

Jails

- For general population needs: one full-time equivalent (FTE) psychiatrist for every 75–100 SMI patients receiving psychotropic medication prescribed for a mental health diagnosis

- For residential treatment units or the equivalent (where a mental health diagnosis is a requirement for admission): one FTE psychiatrist for every 50 patients

Prisons

- For general population needs: one FTE psychiatrist for every 150–200 SMI inmates receiving psychotropic medication
- For residential treatment units or the equivalent (where a mental health diagnosis is a requirement for admission): one FTE psychiatrist for every 50 patients

It is important to note that these corrections-specific recommendations do not apply to other types of community or institutional facilities, where different degrees of acuity and varying patient needs may require different levels of staffing.

Many correctional facilities and systems require remedial efforts. Additional psychiatric time will be necessary for staff education and training, to establish needed linkages with outpatient providers, to review and revise formularies, and for other quality improvement activities.

Education and Training

Professional development for psychiatrists working in correctional facilities is essential. Participation in the educational and training program of the facility and in other continuing medical education activities benefits the facility, the practitioner, and the patients.

Educational and training programs of the facility should include substantial cross-training between custody and clinical staff. Psychiatrists will benefit from training and orientation by custody staff to the correctional culture, including such matters as social order, gang affiliations, risk classification, chain of command, policies on use of force and solitary confinement, management of specific populations, attitudes of correctional officers, and the perceived role of the mental health practitioner in the system. Correctional officers will benefit from training and orientation by clinical staff on such matters as basic mental health principles, signs and symptoms of major mental illness, suicide risk assessment, and violence reduction strategies. Required annual (or more frequent) refresher training courses should supplement mandatory initial training courses.

In addition to intrafacility education and training, psychiatrists should seek additional training from local and national organizations and should be familiar with the relevant literature of the discipline. Training in areas overrepresented in correctional mental health populations (e.g., substance use disorders, trauma, sexual disorders, and personality disorders) is encouraged. Membership in national organizations such as the American Academy of Psychiatry and the Law (AAPL) and the NCCHC offers useful sources of collaboration and support among clinicians working in the field.

Collegial supervision, discussion, and support, along with dedicated time for teaching and mentorship of younger practitioners and trainees, may lessen frustration and burnout and serve as ongoing education. The employment agreement with the facility or system should specifically provide for such activities.

Given the rates of mental illness in correctional facilities, medical schools and psychiatric residencies should provide education and training in correctional psychiatry. The Accreditation Council on Graduate Medical Education already requires that fellowship programs in forensic psychiatry include a substantial experience caring for individuals under correctional supervision. Psychiatrists working in correctional facilities are encouraged to embrace their roles as supervisors and instructors for these trainees. An active liaison and/or affiliation with an academic-medical or other educational institution(s) is advantageous in recruitment, retention, continuing education, career satisfaction, and achievement and maintenance of high-quality services.

Cultural Awareness

Correctional facilities differ from most community settings in gender, racial, ethnic, cultural, and sociodemographic factors. They have high percentages of male inmates, minority ethnic groups, and homeless or impoverished individuals. This contributes to cultural differences among clinical staff, inmates, and security staff. Some psychiatrists practicing in correctional settings have received training outside of the United States, and this may also contribute to important cultural differences. As in any treatment setting, incarcerated individuals deserve equal care regardless of gender, gender preference, racial/ethnic background, socioeconomic status, education, or other cultural factors.

Correctional facilities should provide training to ensure sensitivity to cultural differences and support efforts to overcome impediments to the delivery of mental health services. Such training can foster positive attitudes and acceptance of other cultures by means of didactic and experiential components. The goals and objectives of such training should relate to attitude, knowledge, and skills. Positive attitudes and acceptance of other cultures increase with exposure to and awareness of other belief systems. Desired outcomes include improved acceptance of diverse populations, empathy for the minority experience (including the internalization of experiences of prejudice), and an understanding of concepts of ethnocentric bias and its potential effects.

The general overview of the program should contain information common to minority and ethnic groups and information about the specific ethnic groups with which an individual clinician will most often interface. Themes to pursue may include demographic information and epidemiology, the psychological aspects of immigration, the psychological aspects of minority status, religious and other beliefs and attitudes about psychiatric treatments, sources of misdiagnosis, and frequently misdiagnosed problems. The didactic curriculum should include the presentation of biological, psychological, sociological, economic, ethnic, gender, religious/spiritual, sexual orientation, peer relations, and family factors that significantly influence physical and psychological development (e.g., trauma and juvenile justice exposure).

Informed Consent

Respect for the individual is a core value of the practice of medicine and psychiatry. Obtaining informed and voluntary consent for treatment interventions, regardless of setting, reflects respect and meets the standard of care in psychiatry. The inherently coercive settings of lockups, detention centers, jails, and prisons, by nature of the deprivation of liberty, make it more challenging to obtain voluntary consent, but inmates retain the ability to make treatment decisions within the scope of individual and institutional safety considerations. The principles of informed consent as embodied in the APA's *Principles of Medical Ethics With Annotations Especially Applicable to Psychiatry* (American Psychiatric Association 2013b) remain applicable in correctional facilities. Patients should participate, to the extent possible, in decisions about evaluation and treatment. Psychiatrists should offer to discuss with their patients the nature, purpose, risks, and benefits of treatment options.

Exceptions to the need for informed consent include emergency treatment interventions when obtaining consent is not possible, court-ordered treatment, a patient's knowing waiver of informed consent, and, in very rare and extreme circumstances, therapeutic privilege in the service of avoiding a negative patient outcome. Policies and documentation procedures concerning the right to refuse treatment should conform to the rules and procedures of the jurisdiction in which the facility is located.

Confidentiality and Privacy

Patient privacy in correctional facilities may at times and of necessity be compromised. Nevertheless, the usual principles of confidentiality as embodied in the *Principles of Medical Ethics With Annotations Especially Applicable to Psychiatry* should be goals in the delivery of psychiatric services. This position is supported by the NCCHC's *Standards for Mental Health Services in Correctional Facilities* (National Commission on Correctional Health Care 2008). Very limited modifications may be necessary given institutional security requirements that govern these settings; the responsibilities of the custody staff to protect inmate and staff safety and prevent escape; and the involvement of security staff, at times, in treatment activities (e.g., providing security at the medication window or monitoring outdoor recreation or indoor temperatures for individuals receiving psychotropic medications who may be heat sensitive). Nevertheless, all reasonable efforts should be made to keep patient information confidential. Confidentiality may be particularly important to groups that are frequently encountered in correctional settings and may be at increased risk of victimization from inappropriate disclosure (e.g., persons with HIV/AIDS, persons who have experienced sexual violence, sex offenders, and individuals charged with or convicted of high-profile crimes).

As in the community, psychiatrists working in correctional settings must clearly specify limitations on confidentiality prior to rendering treatment services, except in emergency situations. These limitations for encounters and disclosure include situations when the patient is

- At risk for self-injury or suicide
- At risk for assaultive behavior or committing homicide
- Gravely disabled and unable to care for himself or herself

Additional limitations on confidentiality that may be warranted in a correctional setting include situations when the patient

- Presents a significant risk of escape or threat to the security of the institution, active illicit drug use, or significant contraband use
- Has sustained a serious injury warranting investigation
- Requires coordinated care including movement to a special unit or offsite treatment facility for observation, evaluation, or treatment of an acute psychiatric episode

This list is not meant to be all-inclusive and may be supplemented in accordance with the special needs of each patient or the institution.

The importance of private space for confidential doctor-patient interactions cannot be overstated. Inmates with mental illness may be vulnerable or targeted by other inmates. Without the assurance of privacy, some patients may not seek mental health services or adhere to treatment. However, efforts to speak privately should not be pursued at the risk of reducing patient access to care. For example, a patient may refuse to come out of the cell to attend the clinic for an appointment but may wish to speak with the psychiatrist at cell-side. Psychiatrists need to ensure that such refusals to come out do not arise from external disincentives, such as cell shakedowns occurring during psychiatric appointments. Patients should be encouraged to speak in private settings, but clinicians must use their judgment regarding safety considerations, unit rules, access to treatment, patient wishes, and the therapeutic alliance.

Psychiatrists working in correctional settings may perform non-treatment-related services such as assessments for in-custody disciplinary housing placement. Complex ethical issues arise when a treating psychiatrist participates in the disciplinary process to determine whether a patient should be sanctioned for an infraction or rules violation. If asked to participate, the psychiatrist should obtain the informed consent of the patient and limit involvement solely to providing an opinion on whether there is a psychiatric condition that contributed to the behavior leading to an alleged infraction (i.e., mitigating circumstances) or that is related to the issue of competency to proceed in the disciplinary hearing process. With few exceptions, because of potential conflicting roles, the evaluating clinician should not be the inmate's treating clinician. It is the responsibility of the evaluating psychiatrist to clearly set forth to the inmate any limitations on confidentiality as part of the informed consent process. Treating psychiatrists must not participate in making decisions about discipline, because this crosses ethical boundaries.

Psychiatrists should share relevant confidential information with facility administrators (on a "need to know" basis) when the information has a significant impact on the management of an inmate, safety and security issues, or an inmate's ability to participate in programs. In deciding what information to disclose, it is important that the psychiatrist consider the following:

- The need to balance the therapeutic needs of the patient with the security and stability of the institution
- The challenges inherent in accurately predicting violence and dangerousness, both to self and to others
- The impact of any breach of confidentiality on the relationship with the patient

Psychiatrists working in correctional settings must be able to access patients' relevant community medical and mental health records in order to provide continuity of quality care. The Health Information Portability and Accountability Act (HIPAA) Privacy Rule (45 C.F.R. Subtitle A, §164.512) allows for community providers to provide protected health information without authorization to law enforcement and correctional officials in order to provide health care, maintain inmate and staff safety, and maintain security of the correctional facility.

Psychiatrists must also have efficient access to records from other sites within the same correctional facility (e.g., records from the administrative segregation unit or the infirmary) and communicate relevant confidential information with the consent of the inmate to community providers when the patient is released. Facilities must have mental health record systems that are accessible and comprehensive and support timely service provision.

Psychiatrists in these settings also must be able to provide appropriate information when conducting continuous quality improvement reviews with correctional leadership. This would occur when psychiatrists participate as members of committees such as special needs accommodations, pharmacy and therapeutics, morbidity and mortality, quality improvement, and other related activities.

In light of these special considerations, facilities need written policies on confidentiality and privacy. In facilities where no written policy exists, psychiatrists are encouraged to clarify these issues with the institutional authorities and help develop working policies on the degree to which confidential information can be shared.

Suicide Prevention

The risk of suicide is higher among correctional inmates than among the population at large. Suicide is the leading cause of death in jails and the fifth leading cause of death in prisons (Noonan and Ginder 2013). Suicide risk is also increased in individuals with mental illness, a growing percentage of whom are found in correctional facilities. All nationally recognized correctional mental health standards, including these guidelines, require that each facility have a suicide prevention program for identifying and responding to suicidal inmates.

An inmate may become suicidal at any point during incarceration. High-risk periods include the time of admission, following new legal problems (e.g., new charges, additional sentences, institutional proceedings, denial of parole), following the receipt of bad news (e.g., a serious illness in the family or the loss of a loved one), after a traumatic event (e.g., sexual assault), after experiencing rejection (e.g., by a significant other), or during worsening symptoms of mental illness. Increased suicide risk may also occur during the early phases of recovery from depression or psychotic illness and while the inmate is housed in administrative segregation or other specialized single-cell settings.

Although there are many more suicide attempts and incidents of nonlethal self-harm than completed suicides, any threats of self-harm or self-injurious behavior must be taken seriously. Self-harm behaviors, regardless of motivation, can result in significant morbidity and mortality. For this reason, even behaviors that do not lead to injury should be taken seriously and not dismissed as merely "suicidal gestures."

An adequate suicide prevention program must include the following components, which should be available in a written policy and procedure manual that all staff can easily access:

- Training for all staff who interact directly with inmates to recognize warning signs and intervene appropriately with individuals at risk for suicide
- A formal and detailed suicide risk assessment process
- Identification of inmates at increased risk of suicide through screening at or near the time of admission to the facility and through referral at any time during an individual's incarceration
- An effective and well-understood referral system that allows staff and inmates to bring a suicidal inmate to the prompt attention of a mental health clinician
- Timely evaluation by a mental health clinician to determine the level of risk posed by a referred inmate
- Timely implementation of monitoring interventions such as close observation (at least every 15 minutes), continuous monitoring, alternative housing, or referral to a higher level of care (e.g., infirmary or hospital). When indicated, a psychiatrist–either via phone call or in person–should assist in the decision about interventions. Any mental health clinician may order an increase in monitoring level, but a decrease in level may be ordered only by a psychiatrist or doctoral-level mental health clinician after an in-person evaluation.
- Housing options that allow for adequate monitoring of suicidal inmates by staff. Suicidal inmates should not be placed in isolation settings without continuous monitoring. Continuous monitoring for active suicidality should occur regardless of housing location. Supervision aids such as video monitoring may be used as a supplement to, but not as a replacement for, active staff monitoring.

- Communication among mental health, correctional, medical, and other staff of the specific needs and risks presented by a suicidal inmate
- Timely provision of mental health services, including medication, individual and group therapies, and crisis intervention, for chronically or acutely suicidal inmates
- Accurate, behaviorally specific, and highlighted documentation in the medical record of behaviors or statements that indicate suicide risk
- Quality improvement reviews with psychiatric staff participation of suicide attempts and completed suicides to help prevent future occurrences
- Critical incident support, opportunities for peer-to-peer discussion, and availability of Employee Assistance Program support for completed suicides to assist staff and inmates in dealing with feelings of guilt, fear, grief, and anger

Mental Health Treatment

Constitutional and statutory law, and these guidelines, requires that all inmates have timely and effective access to mental health treatment regardless of where they are housed. Faced with the risk of costly and time-consuming litigation, correctional leaders have increasingly opted for compliance with national health standards and achieving accreditation (Anno 2001; Rold 2008). Jails, prisons, juvenile detention, and other correctional facilities may be accredited by the NCCHC (an offshoot of the American Medical Association), the Joint Commission, the American Correctional Association, or a combination of these. Since 2008, the NCCHC has published standards specifically for mental health services (National Commission on Correctional Health Care 2008). These parallel the standards for health services in jails (National Commission on Correctional Health Care 2014a) and prisons (National Commission on Correctional Health Care 2014b) in format and substance but explicitly specify the standards for adequate delivery of mental health services in nine general areas: governance and administration, safety, personnel and training, health care services and support, inmate care and treatment, health promotion, special mental health needs and services, clinical records, and medical-legal issues. Although national accreditation is typically voluntary, it is often a contractual requirement for universities, other health care systems, and private vendors who provide mental health care services to correctional systems. In addition, when facilities undergo investigation or litigation or are placed under federal oversight, they are often mandated to establish and maintain national accreditations. In this section of the principles governing the delivery of psychiatric services in correctional facilities, we seek to clarify the purposes of such treatment and the modalities that may be employed.

The principles and guidelines for psychiatric services in correctional facilities outlined herein seek to ensure that inmates have such access to care to meet their serious mental health needs. The parameters of access to care include an identified responsible mental health authority; appropriate screening, referral, mental health evaluation, and treatment; clinical autonomy; and ensuring that mental health services are coordinated and delivered in an effective, safe, timely, and responsive fashion. This requires establishing and implementing policies for clinical aspects of the mental health program; monitoring the appropriateness, timeliness, and responsiveness of mental health care and treatment; and ensuring appropriate follow-up (National Commission on Correctional Health Care 2008, 2014a, 2014b). Administrative decisions (such as utilization review) are coordinated, if necessary, with clinical needs so that patient care is not jeopardized. Finally, custody and administrative staff support and do not interfere with the implementation of clinical decisions and treatment services.

Mental health treatment in the correctional setting, like that in any setting, is defined as the use of a variety of mental health therapies, including biological, psychological, and social therapies, to alleviate symptoms that cause distress or interfere with a person's ability to function. An additional and unique dimension within corrections is the need for timely communication about a patient's mental health needs with other clinical and nonclinical staff. This communication with nonclinical staff may seem counterintuitive to psychiatrists and other mental health staff who are well versed in the need for privacy of protected health information and the confidential nature of mental health treatment. Privacy and confidentiality concerns may result in reluctance to share vital information with non–health care staff. Information about an inmate's significant mental health needs, however, has relevance to correctional classification, housing, work and program assignments, admissions to and transfers from institutions, transportation, disciplinary measures and proceedings, and other custodial decisions (Appelbaum et al. 2001). Communicating this information helps preserve the health and safety of that inmate, other inmates, and staff while maintaining the correctional system's primary focus and need for custody and control. Mental health treatment involves more than just prescribing psychotropic medication, and psychiatrists should not be limited to this role.

The fundamental policy goal for correctional mental health treatment is to provide timely access to mental health services to all inmates who need them, wherever they are housed. Inmates must have access to appropriate mental health treatment that is equivalent to that which is available in the community. Furthermore, patient autonomy generally requires that inmates, in consultation with QMHPs, make their own decisions regarding their mental health care. The purposes of mental health treatment in correctional settings include

- Relieving suffering and impairment caused by mental illness
- Enhancing safety for the inmate and others
- Improving the inmate's ability to participate in educational, treatment, and other programs offered

In pretrial settings, treatment might include a jail-based restoration-of-competency program or transfer to an off-site forensic unit or state hospital for restoration of competency to stand trial. The return of the inmate from the off-site forensic psychiatric setting may pose challenges regarding continuity of care and medication adherence. In a correctional setting, the inmate might return to a general-population housing setting with the ability to participate in programs, including suitable outpatient mental health programs, and preparation for release. Another placement might be to transition an inmate with a chronic mental illness who has achieved clinical stabilization within an intensive psychiatric unit setting to a less restrictive "sheltered" or specialized mental health housing treatment program within the correctional environment.

Treatment modalities should be provided in a way that is consistent with generally accepted psychiatric practices and with institutional requirements. Examples of specific psychiatric treatment services include psychiatric diagnostic evaluation, case consultation, and medication treatment services. Examples of other mental health treatment services include the development of a continuum of mental health screening and triage, outpatient, inpatient, crisis management, and specialized programs as needed. Psychoeducation (education about mental illnesses and management) and skills training are additional important mental health treatment components. Nationwide implementation of the Prison Rape Elimination Act of 2003 (Public Law 108-79) is now generating mental health and medical referrals of offenders who disclose past or recent victimization and/or perpetration of sexual abuse. The final rule on implementation guidelines was published in 2012 (U.S. Department of Justice 2012).

Many correctional adaptations of disease-specific protocols now exist. These rely on nationally promulgated evidence-based disease management guidelines, clinical guidelines, and position statements from organizations such as the NCCHC and the Society of Correctional Physicians. A *clinical guideline* is a consensus statement designed to help practitioners and their patients make decisions about appropriate health care for specific clinical circumstances. Clinical guidelines contain up-to-date information and evidence-based recommendations on best practices for the clinical management of specific medical and mental health conditions. The application of guidelines nevertheless requires clinical judgment because some situations may appropriately fall outside of guideline boundaries.

Referral for Mental Health Treatment

Referral is the process by which an individual is provided the opportunity for a mental health evaluation. Referrals may be generated through reception screening, mental health intake screening, or later processes (including self-referral; referral by custody or other clinical staff; concerns raised by other offenders; or requests from family members, judges, lawyers, or legislative staff). As noted earlier, referrals must be timely, be reviewed by a clinician, receive a professional clinical judgment, and deliver the care that is ordered (National Commission on Correctional Health Care 2008, 2014a, 2014b).

The referral process may be simple or complex, depending on the policies and procedures, size and type of facility, clinical urgency of the situation, and available mental health coverage. The referral process should be specifically defined and the roles of the participants clearly delineated.

Referrals should be time constrained: a maximum time for response to each referral, suitable to the situation (i.e., routine, urgent, emergent), should be set out in the facility's operating standards. Timely referral and response should be designated as indicators of quality care. Whenever possible, a continuous quality improvement program monitors and improves mental health care delivered in the facility.

Mental Health Evaluations

The nature and characteristics of mental health evaluations depend on context. In a lockup setting, where the major focus may be the timely identification and transfer of an inmate with SMI to a designated correctional psychiatric unit or an off-site psychiatric facility, evaluations tend to be more brief and focused. In a jail or prison setting that has additional levels of mental health housing and treatment services or alternative off-site arrangements, evaluations and interventions may be more detailed and extensive. At a minimum, a mental health evaluation includes information related to current symptomatology, past treatment, suicide and violence risk, current medications, comorbid medical problems, and substance use.

Therapeutic Milieu

To the extent possible, mental health treatment should be provided in a setting that is conducive to the achievement of its goals. This includes the physical setting and the social-emotional setting, in which an atmosphere of empathy and respect for the dignity of the patient is maintained. Mental health services are conducted in private and carried out in a manner that encourages the patient's subsequent use of services. A therapeutic milieu implies the following conditions:

- A sanitary and humane environment
- Written procedures
- Adequate medical and mental health staffing
- Adequate allocation of resources for the prevention of suicide, self-injury, and assault
- Adequate observation, treatment, and supervision
- Social interactions that foster recovery

Providing privacy for mental health services and cell-side mental health encounters is a special challenge. According to the NCCHC Mental Health Standards (National Commission on Correctional Health Care 2008), when the patient poses a probable risk to the safety of staff or others, security personnel must be present. Nevertheless, adequate privacy should be provided (e.g., use of a programming cell). The patient-psychiatrist relationship may be eroded if privacy is not provided during clinical encounters. Mental health triage commonly occurs at cell-side. If the triage discussion becomes more involved, the clinician should maintain privacy by moving the patient to a clinical setting.

Transfer to a correctional mental health unit or off-site mental health facility must be available when it is clinically indicated. As safety and security allow, self-help and peer support programs or activities that contribute to the overall goals of the mental health services should be promoted and encouraged by clinical staff.

Levels of Care

Mental health services are generally provided in a continuum of treatment settings or levels of care. These levels of care include outpatient, residential, crisis intervention, infirmary, and inpatient services. Outpatient treatment is the least intensive level. Patients live in a general population housing unit with other inmates, many of whom do not need psychiatric care. Residential treatment programs are more intensive and usually exist in dedicated housing. As with similar programs in the community, residential treatment is provided for patients with chronic and serious mental illness who do not require acute care but do need enhanced services. These designated housing units provide a therapeutic environment for those patients who may not function adequately in the general population.

Crisis intervention includes supervised stabilization and/or diagnostic assessment, often in an infirmary setting, and short-term counseling. A psychiatric inpatient program is the most intensive level of care. Many systems provide this through collaboration with a local or state psychiatric hospital.

Community Reentry Planning

There is increased recognition of the risk for reincarceration of individuals with SMI (Baillargeon et al. 2009). Timely and effective discharge planning is essential to continuity of care and an integral part of adequate mental health treatment. This is true whether the patient is released into the community or transferred to another correctional facility. Because discharges (e.g., from jails) or transfers (e.g., between prisons) may occur on short notice, discharge planning needs to begin as part of the initial treatment plan. Discharge planning is provided for all inmates with serious mental health needs as well as other mental health caseload inmates whose release is imminent, although the nature of the discharge planning process will vary on the basis of the inmate's needs. For planned discharges, health care or other designated staff should arrange for a sufficient supply of current psychotropic medications to last until the patient can be seen by a community health care provider. Patients with critical medical and/or mental health needs must have appointments scheduled with community providers, including arrangements for psychiatric hospitalization as needed (National Commission on Correctional Health Care 2008, 2014a, 2014b). Confidentiality concerns should be addressed to facilitate sharing of information among providers in different settings.

In Part 2 of these guidelines, we list essential services for community reentry planning. These include assessments, appointments, and linkages to community-based services. In addition, reentry planning may include help with obtaining financial benefits (e.g., Medicaid) and housing (because of the high incidence of homelessness in correctional populations). Finally, it is recommended that the family and other community-based resources and supports, when available, be included in the community reentry planning process.

Ethical Issues

Ethical issues have particular concern for psychiatrists practicing in correctional facilities because of the inherently coercive environments and the pervasiveness of complex problems of dual loyalty. The terms *dual loyalty* or *dual agency* describe those situations in which a psychiatrist is subject to more than one authority or moral principle. Correctional psychiatrists sometimes face conflicts between two distinct roles and responsibilities: those as the patient's treating physician versus those as an employee or agent of the correctional facility. Conflicts can arise when the psychiatrist's duties to the patient clash with duties to the correctional organization. Evaluations for legal purposes (e.g., competence to stand trial, parole eligibility, or responsibility for disciplinary infractions) present heightened conflicts for a treating psychiatrist. Forensic and clinical roles have different professional responsibilities and ethical duties. NCCHC accreditation standards explicitly prohibit health care workers from collecting forensic information (National Commission on Correctional Health Care 2014b, p. 149). Although NCCHC standards make an exception for court-ordered psychiatric or psychological evaluations with the informed consent of the inmate, we recommend that psychiatrists not conduct court-ordered evaluations for the patients they treat or have treated. A mental health professional who has no treatment relationship with the inmate may conduct these evaluations in settings that require staff to do them. The earlier section "Confidentiality and Privacy" reviews psychiatrist involvement in the disciplinary process.

In the introduction to the first edition of these guidelines (American Psychiatric Association 1989), we noted that "the psychiatrist practicing in these settings is *always* bound by the standards of professional ethics as set out in the APA's *Annotations Especially Applicable to Psychiatry to the AMA's Principles of Medical Ethics*. These are the most fundamental statements of the moral and ethical foundations of professional psychiatric practice" (p. 5). That document's latest edition (American Psychiatric Association 2013b) continues to have only two annotations that specifically apply to psychiatrists practicing in a criminal justice setting. The first annotation relates to a period of time very early in the criminal justice process: before an individual has been arraigned. Annotation 13 to Section 3 of the *Principles of Medical Ethics With Annotations Especially for Psychiatry* (American Psychiatric Association 2013b) states that "ethical considerations in medical practice preclude the psychiatric *evaluation* of any person charged with criminal acts prior to access to, or availability of, legal counsel. The only exception is the rendering of care to the person for the sole purpose of medical *treatment*." It is significant to note that here, too, at the very beginning of the legal process—even before the arraignment process—there is a distinction made between a treating responsibility and an evaluation obligation. The point is that before a person who has been arrested has been before a judge (and until that person is able to speak to a lawyer and informed of the charges and apprised of his or her rights), a forensic psychiatric *evaluation* should not be performed.

The only other annotation relating to correctional psychiatry relates to a time at the end of the criminal justice process: when the inmate is to be executed. Annotation 4 of Section 1 of the *Principles of Medical Ethics With Annotations Especially for Psychiatry* states that "a psychiatrist should not be a participant in a legally authorized execution." Here, too, it seems that a distinction is being drawn between the psychiatrist's responsibility to treat the inmate (and the responsibility to benefit the patient) and a duty or responsibility to the state.

The AAPL has addressed matters relating to correctional psychiatry in more detail. Under the heading of confidentiality, *The Ethics Guidelines for the Practice of Forensic Psychiatry* (American Academy of Psychiatry and the Law 2005) state that

> in a *treatment* situation, whether in regard to an inpatient or to an outpatient in a parole, probation, or conditional release situation, the psychiatrist should be clear about any limitations on the usual principles of confidentiality in the *treatment* relationship and assure that these limitations are communicated to the patient. The psychiatrist should be familiar with the institutional policies in regard to confidentiality. Where no policy exists, the psychiatrist should clarify these matters with the institutional authorities and develop working guidelines to define his role. (*emphasis added*)

With regard to consent, the AAPL Ethics Guidelines state that "consent to *treatment* in a jail or prison or other criminal justice setting must be differentiated from consent to *evaluation*. The psychiatrists providing treatment in these settings should be familiar with the jurisdiction's rules in regard to the patient's right to refuse treatment" (American Academy of Psychiatry and the Law 2005). Then, more broadly, the guidelines state that "a *treating* psychiatrist should generally avoid agreeing to be an expert witness or to perform an *evaluation of his patient for legal purposes* because a *forensic evaluation* usually requires that other people be interviewed and testimony may adversely affect the therapeutic relationship." Here, too, a clear distinction is made between treatment and evaluation.

Finally, we note that there is one code of ethics that seeks to apply ethical principles specifically to clinical practice in correctional settings: that of the American Correctional Health Services Association (1990). Although the association's Code of Ethics does not explicitly distinguish between treatment and evaluation functions, this distinction is implicit in three separate sections: the collection and analysis of specimens for diagnostic purposes only; the performance of body cavity searches only by correctional health professionals not in a provider/patient relationship; and the injunction to honor custody procedures but not participate in actions such as inmate escort, security supervision, or strip searches (American Correctional Health Services Association 1990).

Hunger Strikes

Hunger strikes in prisons and detention facilities (especially those that house illegal immigrants or political prisoners) have become more common in the United States and around the world. Hunger strikes are considered a medical emergency, and psychiatrists are often asked to evaluate inmates to determine if they have the mental capacity to make an informed decision regarding continuation of the hunger strike (Daines 2007). Psychiatrists can perform evaluations to rule out underlying mental illness as a cause of the hunger strike (e.g., suicidal depression or delusions regarding prison food). There is currently no consensus to guide psychiatrists in the United States on the ethical standards of force-feeding to end hunger strikes in correctional facilities (Crosby et al. 2007; Keram 2015). Although the World Medical Association and the American Medical Association, with limited exceptions, have taken stands against the practice (Lazarus 2013; World Medical Association 2006), the Supreme Court of Connecticut, in *Commissioner of Correction v. Coleman* (303 Conn. 800 38 A. 3d 84 [2012]), found that the state's interest in the inmate's health and legitimate penological interests in the safety of the facility outweighed the inmate's right to autonomy. Furthermore, the court ruled that force-feeding did not violate constitutional rights to free speech and privacy.

Research

Research provides the basis for development of best practices and quality care standards for patients. Psychiatric research contributes to the community at large by investigating methods to improve treatment outcomes for offenders with mental illness. Psychiatric research may assist mental health practitioners in their clinical work and help inmate patients. Other types of research design, including epidemiological and noninvasive studies, can yield useful information about the precursors of mental illness in offenders, incidence and prevalence of mental illness, program design, physical plant design, and planning for services. However, research with prisoners as subjects requires special legal safeguards and clinical considerations.

In addition to usual precautions for patients in studies, researchers must provide extra safeguards for inmates because incarceration is an inherently coercive setting that undermines an inmate's ability to provide freely given informed consent for participation in research. As a result of significant rights violations in the use of prisoners as research subjects in the United States in the wake of World War II, the U.S. Code of Federal Regulations (CFR) has a section for the protection of human subjects in research (Title 45, Part 46) specifically dedicated to the protection of prisoners (U.S. Department of Health and Human Services 2009). Subpart C, which has not changed significantly since the late 1970s, highlights four areas of acceptable research on prisoners: 1) the study of the possible causes, effects, and processes of incarceration and of criminal behavior; 2) the study of prisons as institutional structures or of prisoners as incarcerated persons, provided that the study presents no more than minimal risk or inconvenience; 3) the study of conditions particularly affecting prisoners as a class (e.g., alcoholism, drug abuse, sexual assault); and 4) research on practices, both innovative and accepted, that have the intent and reasonable probability of improving the health or well-being of the subject. The guidelines set forth in the CFR should be strictly observed for any projects receiving federal funding. The majority of state-sponsored and academic institutions also follow similar guidelines, and these guidelines should be observed. All pharmacological research must comply with U.S. Food and Drug Administration regulations that control the conduct of drug trials with prison populations.

For psychiatrists interested in research or results of research in this population, more resources are now available. More governmental and philanthropic organizations now recognize the benefit and results of research in the appropriate and timely treatment of this population. Organizations such as the Council of State Governments, the Academic Consortium on Criminal Justice Health, and the Academic and Health Policy Conference on Correctional Health provide forums for presentation and encouragement of research in this area.

Administrative Issues

Access to mental health services in correctional settings requires a balance between security and treatment needs. There is no fundamental incompatibility between security and treatment. It should be universally recognized that good treatment can contribute to good security, and good security can contribute to good treatment (Appelbaum et al. 2001).

Health Services Administration

The effective provision of mental health services requires integration of mental health administration into the overall management of the facility. Close integration of clinical, substance abuse, and security services fosters comprehensive treatment.

A qualified health care administrator with a sound clinical background should have supervisory authority over professionals who work with mental health patients and specified authority over security staff on specialized mental health units. Mental health administrative personnel need written policies on critical issues such as staffing patterns, admission, referral, discharge criteria, health care management, information management, and interagency and intra-agency communications, especially on confidential medical and mental health information.

Psychiatrists can provide administrative leadership and clinical care. Even when control may be in the hands of nonpsychiatrists, attention to quality care serves the best interests of the patient.

Relationship With Custody Administration

Mental health professionals require training in and understanding of security needs and issues. Clinical leadership and sufficient staffing and resources help create an environment that promotes therapeutic interactions. The same occurs with good working relationships among all disciplines (e.g., nurses, psychologists, psychiatrists, social workers, correctional officers, and correctional counselors), especially when an administrator with clinical experience serves as the coordinator for mental health disciplines. Clinical input also has value regarding decisions about work and housing assignments and institutional transfers.

Mental health professionals work within their professional scope of practice as defined in that jurisdiction's licensure process (usually by the state) and within the bounds of training, expertise, and skills. As such, mental health professionals provide services within a standard of care. However, chronic shortage of professional resources is a common problem in correctional settings. At the very least, a psychiatrist's responsibility includes communicating shortcomings and resource needs to the appropriate authority.

Mental health staff need knowledge about and sensitivity to the concerns of security staff. They get information about security through education and training for working in these settings. Similarly, organized programs can teach and train custody personnel about mental health issues. Programs that especially benefit from carefully administered integration include those on developmental disabilities, neurological impairments, alcohol and drug abuse, and sex offenses.

Interprofessional Relationships

Delivery of mental health services in correctional settings requires cooperation by all professionals, including psychiatrists, psychologists, social workers, nurses, other health care staff, correctional counselors, and correctional officers. The manner in which these professionals interact is critical to provision of care. Psychiatrists working in correctional institutions need to recognize the importance of safety and security of inmates and staff. Interprofessional relationships may become strained if mental health or medical interventions conflict with correctional practices.

Mental health services require strong leadership. Facilities that have only one or two clinicians on staff and where crisis intervention is the primary mode of mental health service provision still need a supervisor, even if he or she is not located on site. Facilities with several mental health staff members and different levels of mental health care can have a designated mental health administrator who understands the interprofessional roles of custody, medical, and mental health staff. The mental health administrator functions as a leader to oversee the development of mental health policies and procedures that are coordinated with custody's policies and medical services. Good mental health leaders communicate well among custody, medical, and mental health staffs. They become the conduit for all interprofessional relationships that affect delivery of services. They solve problems and compromise in difficult situations without sacrificing the care of the patient. Doing this requires a healthy respect for the correctional environment and the challenges faced by correctional professionals.

Thoughtful mental health professionals respect each other's expertise and contributions and work well together. They consult on a formal and informal basis and share their special skills in an atmosphere of mutual confidence and trust. The mental health administrator serves a crucial role in assuring that all mental health professionals work together as a team.

Supervisory Roles

Administrative supervision and clinical supervision of staff require different types of expertise. Not all psychiatrists have administrative expertise. Administrative issues, such as inmate housing and on-call coverage, sometimes impinge on clinical decision making. Correctional settings use different models of supervision. Regardless of the model used, psychiatrists have a major role to play in supervising delivery of mental health services, and they retain professional independence for their clinical decisions.

Jail Diversion and Alternatives to Incarceration

More than 500,000 persons with SMIs are admitted to U.S. jails each year. Mental health diversion programs designed to transfer people from the criminal justice system to community-based mental health and substance abuse services are growing in number. There are two types of diversion programs: prebooking and postbooking. *Prebooking* programs involve police and emergency mental health responses that provide alternatives to booking people with mental illness into jail. *Postbooking* programs generally comprise three subtypes: 1) dismissal of charges in return for agreement to participate in a negotiated set of services, 2) deferred prosecution with requirements for treatment participation, and 3) postadjudication release in which conditions for probation include requirements for mental health and substance abuse services.

Some individuals with mental illness must be held in jail because of the seriousness of the alleged offense and/or their histories of nonappearance in court. They need access to mental health treatment within the jail. However, many individuals with less serious, nonviolent crimes can safely be diverted from jail to community-based mental health programs.

People who receive mental health treatment in the community usually have a better long-term prognosis and less chance of returning to jail for a similar offense than people who do not receive mental health treatment. In addition, diversion of individuals with mental illnesses from the criminal justice system helps promote smooth jail operations.

The best diversion programs view detainees as citizens of the community who require a broad array of services, including mental health care, substance abuse treatment, housing, and social services. They recognize that some individuals come into contact with the criminal justice system because of fragmented services, the nature of their illnesses, and the lack of social support and other resources. They know that people should not be detained in jail simply because they have a mental illness. Only diversion programs that address this fragmentation by integrating an array of mental health and other support services, including case management and housing, can break the unproductive cycle of decompensation, disturbance, and arrest.

PART 2

Guidelines for Psychiatric Services in Correctional Facilities

Introduction

The following guidelines for psychiatric services in correctional facilities are based on the principles governing the delivery of psychiatric services presented in Part 1 of this document. Part 3 applies these guidelines to special populations of inmates. These guidelines supplement, but do not replace, the standards developed by the National Commission on Correctional Health Care (NCCHC). The broad outline of these guidelines includes three basic types of services: 1) screening, referral, and evaluation; 2) treatment; and 3) community reentry planning.

Reception Mental Health Screening and Referral

All newly admitted inmates have a reception (or receiving) mental health screening within 4 hours of arrival at a facility. Most facilities follow written protocols and procedures and use a standardized form to document information and observations. In smaller facilities this information may be gathered by a correctional officer with additional health training. Larger facilities may use registered nurses or other health professionals with additional mental health training. All health encounters other than general rounds should be conducted in private settings. Mental health professionals who have safety concerns can request a correctional officer to stand at a reasonable distance outside of a partially open door or, if necessary, to be present in the room during the examination. Facilities can require that all custody staff sign confidentiality agreements at the time of their employment and that initial and annual mental health training of all staff include reviews of guidelines on confidentiality of inmate health information. Inmates with abnormal behaviors or positive findings on the reception mental health screening need triaged referrals for further evaluation, on either an emergent or urgent basis, with time frames defined by policy.

Essential Components

- The screening occurs within 4 hours of the inmate's arrival.
- Screening includes observation and structured inquiry into mental health history and symptoms, including questions about suicide history, ideation, and potential; prior psychiatric hospitalizations and treatment; and current and past medications, both prescribed and actually taken.
- Screening may be conducted by the booking officer, other custody personnel, supervisors, or medical intake nurse. The screener must have training in mental health screening and referral. For jails, lockups, and detention centers, information about the inmate's behavior leading up to and during the arrest should be obtained from the arresting officer if available.
- Referrals should be made for emergent or urgent evaluations for inmates with findings.
- Referral to nursing staff should be made for inquiry about reported active prescriptions. Correctional facilities can verify prescriptions by calling the prescribing agency, pharmacy, or sending facility and obtain bridging medication orders for inmates until they can be seen and assessed by an authorized prescriber.
- A standardized procedure should be used, with observations and responses documented on a standard form in the permanent health record.
- Policies and procedures should specify required actions and time frames after positive screening findings.
- Psychiatrists may have limited roles in direct provision of this service and may participate in the following activities:
  a. Development of screening forms and procedures
  b. Training officers and health care personnel to use the screening instrument and to make appropriate referrals
  c. Development of written referral procedures for inmates identified during the screening as being at high risk
  d. Monitoring the quality of the intake process, including efficacy of identification of inmates needing referral and timeliness of referrals
  e. Prescribing appropriate verified medications, or reasonable formulary substitutions, and monitoring laboratory studies until the patient can be seen, customarily within 10 business days for nonacute issues and sooner if clinically indicated

Intake Mental Health Screening and Referral

Intake mental health screening is defined as a more comprehensive examination of each newly admitted inmate within 14 days of arrival at an institution. It includes a review of the reception mental health screening, medical screening, behavioral observation, review of mental health history, assessment of suicide potential, and mental status examination. Frequently, detainees are booked into jails late at night and while intoxicated. They often give negative responses to questions on the receiving screening in order to speed up the booking process. In prisons, similar issues may occur because of inmate anxiety in a new setting. The intake mental health screening can reveal chronic medical and mental health problems that were not reported on entry into the facility and lead to referrals to chronic care clinics or mental health clinics to ensure identification and treatment of the inmate's health issues.

Essential Components

- The screening is conducted by a qualified mental health professional (QMHP) privileged for independent assessment on the basis of discipline-specific professional standards and state statutes.
- A standardized procedure should be used, with observations and responses documented in the permanent health record.
- Policies and procedures specify required actions and time frames after positive screening observations.
- The inmate is given detailed information about access to mental health services.
- The psychiatrist generally has a limited role in the direct provision of this service but may participate in the following activities:
  a. Development of intake mental health screening forms and informational material
  b. Training health care staff to use intake mental health screening forms and informational (orientation) materials
  c. Developing written referral procedures for inmates identified as requiring mental health evaluation
  d. Monitoring the quality of the referral process to a mental health professional or psychiatrist and whether identification and referral assessments are timely

Postclassification Referral

The initial classification gathers information needed to assign inmates to appropriate housing and programs. Inmates not referred during receiving or intake mental health screening may subsequently need mental health services. *Postclassification referral* is defined as the process by which such individuals are brought to the attention of mental health staff for brief mental health assessment or comprehensive mental health evaluation.

Essential Services

- The referral process may be simple or complex, depending on the facility, the urgency of the situation, and the mental health coverage provided. Facility mental health services plans include written procedures for these referrals.
- Mental health emergency services must be accessible on referral on a 24-hour basis.
- Inmates awaiting emergent or urgent mental health evaluation or transfer may require special safety precautions, including continuous observation or staggered observation at least every 15 minutes, often conducted by security staff, until the evaluation or transfer occurs.
- Training of health care and custody staff occurs at time of hire and during annual updates and includes how and when to use the referral process.
- Inmates receive timely orientation and explanation of the referral process.
- Psychiatrists assist in developing referral policies and procedures and in training staff in the use of the referral system.

Routine Segregation Clearance and Rounds

Segregation is a high-risk housing area in which a disproportionate number of completed suicides occur compared with general housing units. Inmates may be placed in segregation for protective custody, disciplinary infractions, or administrative reasons (e.g., affiliation with a gang, assault history). Prior to placing inmates in segregation, facilities need to provide mental health screening that includes a suicide risk assessment and a determination of whether the inmate's serious mental illness is likely to worsen in this environment. Smaller facilities usually provide only a nursing assessment, but those with sufficient mental health staff use a QMHP to complete these assessments. In addition, facilities provide nursing rounds and mental health rounds with a frequency determined by the degree of isolation of inmates. These rounds increase access to health services for the segregated inmate and monitor for signs of decompensation (see Appendix). Please refer to the section "Mental Illness and Segregation" in Part 3 for additional guidance.

Essential Services

- A registered nurse or a QMHP (when available) usually performs the preplacement assessment.
- Medical or mental health staff conduct segregation rounds at least weekly for inmates who have regular access to social contacts. Inmates in extreme isolation need at least daily medical rounds and weekly mental health rounds.
- Psychiatrists can participate in quality improvement projects on segregation rounds and provide supervision and training to mental health staff who conduct rounds to ensure completion of appropriate risk assessments. Psychiatrists are encouraged to periodically participate in the mental health rounds to be familiar with the setting and establish a positive presence with both inmates and custody staff.

Brief Mental Health Assessment

A *brief mental health assessment* is defined as a mental health examination appropriate to the level of services needed.

Essential Services

- Brief mental health assessments occur within 72 hours of a positive screening and referral. Urgent cases receive immediate evaluation after referral. Each individual whose screening reveals mental health problems has a brief mental health assessment in an office with sound privacy whenever possible, with a written recommendation for a comprehensive mental health evaluation and treatment if indicated (see next section). When clinically appropriate, an individual may be referred directly for a comprehensive mental health evaluation without a brief mental health assessment.
- The findings of brief mental health assessments are documented in the confidential health record.
- Trained and privileged mental health professionals conduct the brief mental health assessment, which includes a mental status examination, diagnostic formulation, recommendations, and treatment plan if indicated.
- Psychiatrists can have a direct or indirect role in providing this service, including

   a. Development of policies and procedures
   b. Performing the mental health evaluation or consultation
   c. Supervision and training of the mental health staff

Comprehensive Mental Health Evaluation

A *comprehensive mental health evaluation* consists of a face-to-face interview in an office with sound privacy and a review of available health care records and collateral information. It concludes with a diagnostic formulation and, at least, an initial treatment plan.

Essential Services

- A comprehensive mental health evaluation occurs when the brief mental health assessment is not adequate.
- The time frame for completion of the comprehensive mental health evaluation depends on level of urgency.
- The findings of the comprehensive mental health evaluation are documented in the confidential health record.
- Psychiatrists or other appropriately licensed or credentialed mental health professionals conduct the comprehensive mental health evaluation.
- Psychiatrists can have a direct or indirect role in providing this service, including the following:

  a. Performing all or part of the comprehensive mental health assessment when appropriate or necessary (e.g., when an inmate is taking psychotropic medications)

  b. Supervision and training of the mental health staff

- Comprehensive mental health evaluations include access to psychological, neuropsychological, medical, laboratory, and neuroimaging services.

Mental Health Treatment

The definition of *mental health treatment* appears in Part 1 of this document. Short-term jail confinements generally emphasize crisis intervention, psychotropic medications, brief or supportive therapies, patient education, and suicide prevention (see "Suicide Prevention" in Part 1). Longer-term jail settings and prisons provide these services plus more extensive treatment services, including verbal therapies and skill-building activities. Use of psychoactive medication requires thoughtful management in correctional settings. Concerns include side-effect management (e.g., heat tolerance, environmental factors, and potential work restrictions) and potential security implications (e.g., diversion or extortion; McKee et al. 2014).

Essential Services

- Mental health treatment includes inpatient care in the correctional facility or in an external hospital.
- The inmate receives 7-day-a-week mental health coverage (including coverage with a board-certified or board-eligible psychiatrist).
- Written treatment plans are provided for each inmate receiving mental health services.
- The facility where the inmate is receiving care has a full range of psychotropic medications with the capacity to administer them, including involuntarily in an emergency where state laws allow.
- Psychotropic medications may be prescribed and are monitored by a psychiatrist or appropriately supervised midlevel prescriber.
- Psychotropic medications are distributed by qualified medical personnel.
- Seven-day-a-week, 24-hour nursing coverage is available in housing areas for inmates with acute or emergent psychiatric problems.
- Special observation, seclusion, and restraint capabilities are available in housing areas for inmates with acute or emergent psychiatric problems.
- Supportive verbal interventions, in an individual or group context, are provided as clinically appropriate.
- Programs that provide productive, out-of-cell activity and teach necessary psychosocial and living skills are offered.
- Training for custody staff in the recognition of mental disorders is provided.

Community Reentry and Transfer Planning

Reentry planning coordinates community-based resources and services for inmates in need of continuing mental health care. In jail settings, continuing needs of inmates at the time of transfer to a prison must be documented and coordinated with the receiving facility. Because of the unpredictability of release or transfer from jail settings, community reentry planning should begin at intake.

Essential Services

- Appointments are arranged with mental health agencies for inmates with serious mental illness, especially those receiving psychotropic medication.
- Arrangements are made with local mental health agencies or prison reception centers to share records, as appropriate, and to have prescriptions renewed or evaluated for renewal.

- Designated staff carry out discharge and referral responsibilities in accordance with the facility's protocol.
- Inmates receiving mental health treatment have assessments for community referral prior to release.
- Prison classification and intake staff are notified of the treatment history and current clinical condition of transferred inmates.
- Whenever possible, service contracts that ensure access to continuity of care in the community are provided.

PART 3

Special Applications of the Principles and Guidelines

Introduction

Some inmate populations have unique evaluation and treatment needs because of their disorders, demographics, or other characteristics. They include individuals with substance use disorders, co-occurring disorders, trauma, nonsuicidal self-injury, infectious diseases, sleep disorders, attention-deficit/hyperactivity disorder (ADHD), and terminal illnesses. They also include females; youths in adult correctional facilities; geriatric persons; lesbian, gay, bisexual, and transgender persons; persons with intellectual or developmental disabilities; and veterans. In this part we address the characteristics that must be considered to ensure access to appropriate mental health services for each of these groups. In this part we also address issues related to segregation, seclusion and restraint, telepsychiatry, and spirituality in the lives of inmates.

Other groups and conditions not addressed herein may also need special clinical policies and procedures developed by psychiatrists. The important issue of mental health services in juvenile correctional facilities requires its own analysis, which is beyond the scope and expertise of this Task Force report.

Treatment Issues: Specific Disorders and Syndromes

Substance Use Disorder

Substance use disorder refers to signs and symptoms (ranked from mild to severe) related to the use of legal and illicit substances such as tobacco and methamphetamine. In the correctional setting, substance use disorders are the most frequently diagnosed mental disorders and often co-occur with serious mental illness (SMI).

More than two-thirds of offenders may have a substance use disorder at the time of their entry into the criminal justice system (Karberg and James 2005). Criminal behavior often occurs when an individual is under the influence of alcohol or other drugs or may be related to efforts to procure or sell substances. Much of the increase in the American prison population is ascribed to criminal activity related to substance use and the implementation of harsher sentencing guidelines for these activities.

Screening and Assessment

Screening for and assessment of substance use disorders, particularly associated intoxication and withdrawal, are critical at entry and transfer to correctional facilities. Although jails and lockups are the point of entry for most individuals entering correctional settings directly from the street, many parole violators proceed directly back to prison. Given the availability of substances of abuse in correctional facilities, individuals transferred between facilities should not be presumed to be drug free.

Screening instruments for substance use may be part of a larger mental health screen or administered separately. Instruments should include, at a minimum, questions about the individual's use of alcohol and other drugs and the patterns of use, with particular attention to signs or symptoms of intoxication or recent use that require a withdrawal protocol. Severe intoxication with some substances (e.g., alcohol, opiates, stimulants) and withdrawal from others (e.g., alcohol, barbiturates, benzodiazepines) can be life threatening and require quick management in collaboration with trained medical staff in a setting appropriate to the acuity.

Jail suicide is closely linked to substance use. Half of all individuals who complete suicide in lockups and detention facilities have a history of substance abuse (Hayes 2010). This number is likely an underestimate because of the limitations of screening procedures. Many of these suicides are related to complications of intoxication or withdrawal. A positive substance intoxication or withdrawal screen should trigger an immediate mental health assessment for suicide risk factors, including mood symptoms and suicidal ideation. Individuals with substance use disorders may also present with medical, neurological, or psychiatric problems. For example, hepatitis, HIV, neuropathies, dementia, and mental illness are frequently comorbid with chronic and/or severe substance use.

Psychiatrists can play an important role in developing the receiving screening instruments; training staff in their use; and educating correctional security, medical, and mental health staff about the signs and symptoms of intoxication and withdrawal.

Diagnosis and Treatment

An evaluation by a psychiatrist or qualified mental health professional (QMHP) helps ensure recognition and management of substance use disorders and avoids misdiagnosing their sequelae as major mental illness (e.g., psychosis as a result of hallucinogen intoxication).

Psychotropic medications prescribed by a psychiatrist or other physician, or another authorized prescriber, may be required during detoxification for management of symptoms associated with withdrawal. Benzodiazepines or methadone/buprenorphine (as appropriate) may help prevent or attenuate withdrawal symptoms, and using them for the short term at tapering dosages lessens the likelihood that the prescribed medication will serve as a substitute for the substance of abuse or be diverted or used inappropriately. Facilities need to avoid formulary restrictions that lead to negative clinical outcomes for patients. Other psychotropic medications, including antipsychotics and mood stabilizers, require judicious use for individuals with no history of mental illness. Such treatment should begin only after detoxification and reasonable substance-free periods. Clinical judgment regarding continuity of care must be used on a case-by-case basis for individuals prescribed psychotropic medications in the community.

Individuals may enter correctional facilities from opioid maintenance programs (e.g., methadone or buprenorphine/naloxone) in the community. Facilities vary in their willingness to continue prescribing these medications, but abrupt cessation or an overly rapid taper must be avoided.

Inmates need access to individualized substance use treatment services, including therapy, group psychotherapy, therapeutic communities, skills training, community support and self-help groups (e.g., Alcoholics Anonymous), and family support. Self-help, 12-step, and peer support groups and networks play an important role in rehabilitation of alcohol and other drug users in the correctional system. Allowing outside community support self-help meetings into the correctional setting permits integration and identification with the community on release.

Rehabilitation takes time and must extend past incarceration in order to have a positive impact on criminal recidivism and the sequelae of substance use. Discharge planning includes referral to community-based substance use treatment services where providers know about the risk of accidental overdose and death for individuals leaving a correctional facility.

Co-occurring Disorders

Co-occurring mental illness and substance use disorders often go undetected in people in contact with the criminal justice system. This failure is typically due to the absence of effective screening and assessment and the difficulty of identifying the often-complicated symptom picture with which this population presents. Nondetection of one or more co-occurring disorders may exacerbate behavior problems, criminogenic risks, and the risk of suicide. Furthermore, it may result in poor outcomes in treatment during incarceration and lead to increased risk of rearrest and reincarceration.

Mental health services in correctional facilities need an integrated and coordinated system of screening, referral, assessment, and diagnosis for co-occurring mental illness and substance use disorders. Such a system should include active collaboration between security staff and treatment staff to share information on signs and symptoms of co-occurring disorders at transition points (e.g., arrest, booking, jail, prison reception) throughout the process. Evidence-based screening tools can help identify individuals who need further assessment. Some screening tools require a clinician to complete, but many can be completed quickly even by nonclinical staff.

Detection of one type of disorder (i.e., substance use or mental illness) should trigger further assessment of the other type of disorder because either can mimic, overshadow, or interfere with detection or affect the presentation of the other.

Persons with co-occurring mental illness and substance use disorders who become justice involved are a particularly service-intensive group. We recommend the following strategies for treating co-occurring disorders. These strategies require adaptation to different settings.

- Integrate treatment that simultaneously addresses mental illness and substance use disorders.
- Treat each disorder as primary, with a simultaneous focus on understanding the interaction.
- Address psychosocial problems and skill deficiencies with individualized programming based on comprehensive assessment and consultation with the patient, treatment provider, and family members (where accessible and with informed consent of the patient).
- Delay starting new psychotropic medications until after detoxification unless it is required by acute symptoms (e.g., psychosis, suicidality).
- Design interventions that differ in intensity, length, and type of services for the particular setting (e.g., prison, jail, or community corrections) and focus on engagement with patients and strength-based, recovery-minded interventions. Extend treatment services into the community, with special attention in discharge planning for co-occurring disorders, housing, employment, and family reconnection.
- Medication-assisted treatment (MAT), when available, can be an effective intervention to help reduce the chance of relapse of the substance use disorder and recidivism, especially when an inmate is close to release.

- Integrate treatment with self-help groups and support networks that can assist treatment participants in maintaining their commitment to daily alcohol and drug abstinence.

Trauma and Posttraumatic Stress Disorder

Traumatic events are widely defined but, according to DSM-5, encompass "exposure to actual or threatened death, serious injury, or sexual violence" (American Psychiatric Association 2013a, p. 271). Exposure can be direct or indirect, as in witnessing an event occurring to another, learning of the event happening to a close friend or family member, or firsthand exposure to disturbing details of the event. Inmates have a high risk for direct and indirect exposure to traumatic experiences (e.g., violence, sexual assault, separation from loved ones) while incarcerated. They also often have developmental histories that include physical, sexual, and emotional abuse and neglect. Rates of current and past traumatic exposure are even higher for individuals with mental illness or substance use disorders in correctional settings. Many of them have experienced chronic stressors such as poverty, homelessness, and social isolation. Individuals with mental illness are more likely to be victimized and to receive additional punishment for rule violations in correctional facilities. Given the risks, rates of posttraumatic stress disorder (PTSD) and many of its complex variants are, not surprisingly, higher in correctional populations than in the general population.

Reactions to trauma, including the development of SMI or PTSD, can significantly affect an incarcerated individual's behavior, medical conditions, response to therapeutic interventions, and risk for violence, self-injury, and suicide. It is therefore important that correctional intake facilities incorporate comprehensive trauma histories into their assessments. Clinicians and custody staff also need training about the impact of trauma and the implications for treatment and management. Because of the high prevalence of lifetime exposure to trauma in correctional populations, particularly physical and sexual abuse, all interventions should involve trauma-informed care, and clinicians need training to assess the psychological consequences of childhood and adult abuse. For example, self-injurious behavior may result from dissociative phenomena or flashbacks of abuse rather than psychotic symptoms or poorly controlled impulsivity.

The use of seclusion, restraint, or forced medication raises special concerns in the context of trauma histories. These methods of control may inadvertently retraumatize inmates who have had similar experiences in the past, both in and out of institutional settings. These measures may be less traumatic if discussions are held with inmates early in their treatment and incarceration. Mental health clinicians can work with patients to develop interventions that will best help calm them down in the event of later agitation. If prophylactic measures are not successful, verbal de-escalation, supportive measures, and recognition of the underlying emotional issues can help avoid use of force.

The use of force is disproportionately used with inmates who are mentally ill. It is increasingly common that mental health staff are requested to attempt face-to-face verbal intervention with inmates prior to the use of calculated (i.e., planned) force with all inmates, especially those with mental illness. Chemical agents (e.g., pepper spray) should rarely be used in health care settings such as infirmaries or special needs units for inmates with mental illness. Psychiatrists may play a key role by participating in staff training in de-escalation techniques.

In addition to training in trauma-informed care and de-escalation techniques, clinicians and custody staff need training about gender differences relevant to the etiology of and response to trauma (Moloney et al. 2009). Studies consistently indicate that incarcerated women have higher rates than men of SMI, substance use disorders, and diagnoses of PTSD (e.g., Fazel and Danesh 2002; Trestman et al. 2007). Women also have higher rates of victimization, including childhood sexual abuse, domestic violence, prostitution-related violence, and sexual assault in correctional settings. Men have perpetrated much of this violence. Wherever possible, same-gender staff should be available, particularly during times of vulnerability (e.g., when inmates are unclothed or are being restrained). Custody and clinical administrators need to ensure that staff responsible for the safety and security of women in correctional facilities minimize the chance of inflicting further trauma.

Incarcerated men have high rates of childhood physical and sexual abuse and direct and indirect exposure to community-related (e.g., gang) and correctional violence. Men and women may respond differently to trauma and to being retraumatized while incarcerated. Women have a higher risk of developing anxiety-related symptoms, sleep disturbances, and PTSD. Men may respond to trauma with more subtle symptoms but may also act out aggressively in response to traumatic triggers. National attention to the importance of trauma sustained in correctional settings, particularly sexual abuse, has increased. The implementation of the Prison Rape Elimination Act (PREA) (U.S. Department of Justice 2012) now generates more medical and mental health referrals and enhances the potential for intervention, support, and treatment for traumatized inmates.

Identifying and treating incarcerated individuals who have symptoms or disorders because of exposure to traumatic events is important for maintaining a safe correctional environment for patients and staff and for preventing criminal and traumatic recidivism upon release. Traumatized individuals, especially those with incarceration histories, are more likely to offend again (e.g., arrests for substance-related crimes, prostitution, or violence) and to return to substance use and less likely to actively engage community mental health resources.

Nonsuicidal Self-Injury

As used in this report, the term *nonsuicidal self-injury* (NSSI) refers to acts intended to cause bodily harm but not death. Such acts include cutting, burning, self-hitting, self-biting, hair pulling, head banging, and ingesting or inserting foreign objects but exclude tattooing, body piercing, risky sexual behaviors, and other behaviors that have nonharmful motivations. Differentiating between NSSI and suicide attempts often poses challenges. Self-reports of intent have limited reliability, and some NSSI behaviors may inadvertently result in death.

Diagnoses commonly associated with NSSI include personality (Cluster B and mixed), mood, psychotic, cognitive, and developmental disorders. The behaviors seen with each condition frequently have distinguishing characteristics (e.g., relief of distress with borderline personality disorder, stereotypic behaviors with intellectual or developmental disorders, and significant tissue damage with psychotic disorders).

NSSI may also occur in the absence of an underlying psychiatric disorder. Interpersonal and environmental factors often trigger and reinforce these behaviors among inmates. Segregation and other lockdown settings have the highest rates, and conflicts with staff or other inmates sometimes precipitate NSSI. Responses that reinforce the behavior can include attention, relief of boredom, change in housing, infirmary or hospital visits, and access to analgesics or other medications. Inmates have limited autonomy, but self-injury offers a way to affect their environment, cope with stress, communicate anger, retaliate against staff by disrupting operations, or meet other needs (Appelbaum et al. 2011).

Labeling and dismissing NSSI as manipulative can be dangerous to the inmate and lead to missed management opportunities. Instead, identification of triggering and reinforcing factors provides the first step toward planning interventions. Such interventions might include creative use of privileges, property, or housing. Effective management always involves shared responsibility and partnership among mental health, medical, and custody personnel.

Psychiatrists must play an active role in addressing NSSI. They can help ensure completion of an adequate diagnostic assessment. Depending on the findings, this may lead to treatment, when appropriate, or working with custody staff to clarify behavioral motivations unrelated to a psychiatric disorder. Psychiatrists can also help develop evidence-based behavioral interventions with realistic goals, such as diminution, but not extinction, in the frequency and severity of NSSI. Accomplishing this requires close collaboration with custody staff and may include explaining the lack of indications for medication or other treatment, acknowledging adverse emotional reactions to the inmate, fostering a dispassionate understanding of the behavioral dynamics, and modeling a professional approach focused on problem solving instead of dominance and control.

Infectious Disease

Adults with mental health and coexisting medical problems are overrepresented in correctional populations. The number of offenders with mental illness and chronic (e.g., cardiac disease, hypertension, diabetes, cancer, end-stage liver and kidney disease) and infectious diseases continues to grow.

HIV and AIDS, hepatitis B and C, tuberculosis, influenza A (H1N1) virus, methicillin-resistant *Staphylococcus aureus*, sexually transmitted diseases (STDs), norovirus, and other gastrointestinal-borne agents are infectious diseases common to correctional settings. HIV and AIDS, viral hepatitis, and tuberculosis, each of which has complex management problems in the community, present even more complicated challenges in correctional settings, including recognizing the need for medical, mental health, and psychiatric services. The risks of social stigma and issues of personal safety complicate confidentiality for the infected inmate, other inmates, and correctional and clinical staff. The usual cultural differences among inmates and security and health care staff may be exacerbated in cases of inmates with these infections, especially HIV/AIDS. Education of staff and inmates about infectious diseases and the means of transmission is especially important for both personal and population health risk reduction. Inmates need access to health educational materials and resources on prevention of transmission and consequences of continued high-risk behaviors for HIV and viral hepatitis such as promiscuity, unprotected intercourse, and intravenous drug use, and prevention of respiratory transmission of tuberculosis.

Correctional facilities that seek accreditation by the National Commission on Correctional Health Care (NCCHC), American Correctional Association, the Joint Commission, or a combination of these routinely monitor for hepatitis, HIV, STDs, and tuberculosis and must have an effective infection control program. For example, the NCCHC has an essential standard requiring the responsible health authority to have a written exposure control plan approved by the responsible physician and reviewed and updated annually.

Inmates need access to mental health treatment regardless of their housing arrangements. Housing restriction (and, particularly in the case of tuberculosis, the need for respiratory isolation) may exacerbate inmates' feelings of abandonment and may lead to a worsening of symptoms of coexisting mental illness.

HIV

Estimated rates of HIV infection in U.S. prison populations have consistently exceeded rates in the general population. There has been a national effort to implement new treatments for HIV, such as combination therapy with multiple antiretroviral drugs, and to develop evidence-based standards of care. These efforts have been highly effective in delaying progression of the disease and transforming HIV into a chronic, manageable condition in most cases. These favorable outcomes come at a price. Medication costs for HIV treatment for prisoners continue to be one of the largest single components of pharmacy expenses for many systems. Further cost increases are expected with the addition of newer classes of antiretroviral drugs.

From a clinical perspective, the most common psychiatric manifestations of HIV/AIDS include early signs of dementia, paranoia, and other psychotic and depressive symptoms. For these reasons, correctional mental health systems might initiate surveillance, outreach programs, or periodic rescreening for early detection and to foster early use of mental health services.

Hepatitis C Virus

Current challenges of hepatitis C virus (HCV) in corrections include the large number of infected offenders, the increased use of medications, and more sophisticated and expensive treatment standards. Several strategies promote uniform, cost-effective processes for managing the often-complex psychiatric and medical needs of HCV-infected offenders. These include chronic care clinics, a case management program, evidence-based disease management guidelines, and formulary controls.

The prevalence of HCV infection is higher among correctional populations than among the general U.S. population (Spaulding et al. 2013). Although most HCV-positive offenders are asymptomatic, those who develop a chronic infection risk serious complications and death. Chronic HCV infection is the leading cause of end-stage liver disease in correctional settings. More cases of liver failure are expected as the proportion of older offenders continues to increase.

HCV-infected offenders who progress to end-stage liver disease require frequent and costly hospitalizations and emergency department services for treatment of bleeding, abdominal fluid retention, and other serious complications. Ultimately, the only viable option for some of these offenders will be liver transplantation, a procedure with substantial initial and subsequent costs. From a clinical perspective, increased ammonia level is commonly associated with behavioral disturbance and presents as a delirium with waxing and waning symptoms that requires timely medical intervention.

Chronic HCV infection is a risk factor for liver cancer and a contributing factor in many liver cancer deaths. Many correctional health care system providers are facing unprecedented challenges in addressing the growing HCV epidemic. These challenges revolve around financial and logistical impediments to evaluating and treating such a large number of HCV-infected offenders along with a constantly evolving consensus about how to best manage the disease in the correctional setting. Meeting these challenges has enormous public health implications because most HCV-infected offenders eventually return to their home communities with the potential to infect others.

Accepted standards of care for the management of HCV infection recommended by the National Institutes of Health and other key groups are rapidly evolving. Until recently, selective treatment with a combination of ribavirin and pegylated interferon to eradicate the virus from the bloodstream and liver biopsy to determine which offenders are most likely to benefit from antiviral therapy was a recommended standard of care. The use of interferon required mental health screening and evaluation when clinically indicated for the development of depressive symptoms and suicidal ideation. This increased the mental health and psychiatric service need demands for correctional facilities. Some systems have limited antiviral treatment options, and some limit treatment to those patients at highest risk for developing cirrhosis and subsequent liver failure.

Offenders with end-stage liver disease and associated conditions are particularly difficult to treat. They may not need medical hospitalization but require specialized housing (often with supplemental oxygen, vital sign and cardiac monitoring, and on-site nursing and medical staff), specialists who can manage end-stage liver disease and associated complications, access to laboratory studies, and coordinated treatment by nursing, medical, psychiatry, and mental health staff.

Many correctional systems struggle to meet the costs of newer HCV medications. Most prison systems treat only a small fraction of infected inmates. Current and emerging therapeutic agents might cure HCV infection in most patients. Mathematical modeling also shows that expanded HCV screening and treatment are cost-effective from the societal perspective (Spaulding et al. 2013). Correctional health leaders and policymakers must carefully weigh the costs of these medications, associated clinical equipment and testing, and staffing. Some newer medications require refrigeration, administration with food, and multiple daily dosing, but other, more costly agents can be administered once a day with purportedly fewer side effects. Some agents require treatment for 24 weeks and rigid compliance for treatment efficacy.

Other chronic infectious diseases present similar challenges for the delivery of psychiatric services, and the principles stated here may also apply to them.

Sleep Disorders

Inmates often seek health care for sleep problems. Although many studies of sleep-wake disorders have been conducted in the general population and different patient groups, studies in correctional settings are limited.

Sleep-wake disorders in DSM-5 include 10 conditions characterized by disturbed sleep and "distress as well as impairment in daytime functioning" (American Psychiatric Association 2013a, pp. 361–422). In the United States, at least 10% of the population has sleep problems (Kraus and Rabin 2012). Of the 10 sleep-wake disorders, insomnia has the most relevance for inmates. It can have serious consequences, such as increased risk of depression and hypertension and impaired daytime functioning.

Acute, short-term insomnia (i.e., less than 3 months) is often caused by situational stress and medical or psychological disorders. Health care personnel need to discuss acute stress with patients and provide appropriate education. Short-term treatment strategies encompass sleep hygiene and, if needed, prescription of sedative-hypnotics, usually a benzodiazepine (Cunnington 2013).

For insomnia disorder (i.e., sleep problems that persist at least 3 nights per week for at least 3 months), empirical evidence supports two treatment strategies. In the past, the predominant approach was pharmacological. However, studies have proven that medication alleviates symptoms for at most the first 6 weeks. Side effects of benzodiazepines include habituation and tolerance, as well as paradoxical effects in the aging population.

Psychological interventions, commonly cognitive-behavioral therapy (CBT), typically yield enduring, clinically significant benefit whether used alone or in combination with pharmacological treatment (Mitchell et al. 2012). CBT for insomnia can be used in individual or group sessions or as self-administered written or audiovisual material. In addition to CBT, sleep hygiene and progressive muscle relaxation have demonstrated efficacy (Morin and Benca 2012).

Some correctional facilities use guidelines to reduce prescriptions of benzodiazepines. Sometimes this results in alternative medications being ordered. These medications can themselves have significant side effects and management concerns.

Insomnia may be related to the conditions of confinement, fears for personal safety with associated hypervigilance, preexisting psychiatric or medical disorders, caffeine intake, drug misuse, lack of physical activity, and daytime napping. Correctional psychiatrists should assess such factors and work to intervene while taking into consideration the possibility of misuse and diversion.

Attention-Deficit/Hyperactivity Disorder

Research suggests that criminal justice populations have an elevated prevalence of ADHD. Although most studies of this population have methodological shortcomings that limit their reliability, ADHD can persist into adulthood and does occur among inmates. Diagnosis and management pose challenges in correctional settings, as they do in the community.

Characteristic symptoms of ADHD such as inattention, restlessness, poor planning, poor frustration tolerance, and impulsivity occur with other psychiatric and medical disorders and as part of ordinary, nonpathological human experience. When due to ADHD, these symptoms have identifiable persistence and severity that significantly disrupt success in social, academic, and vocational areas in both the community and correctional environments. Accurate diagnosis of ADHD generally requires a comprehensive assessment that includes a history of childhood symptoms, review of educational records, use of symptom rating scales, collateral information from reliable third parties who know the patient, and a thorough diagnostic interview with assessment of alternative explanations for the patient's symptoms. Correctional facilities often have limited resources to readily accomplish this detailed assessment.

Along with diagnostic challenges, correctional psychiatrists face obstacles to treating ADHD with standard stimulant medications. The high prevalence of substance use disorders among inmates can lead to false or exaggerated presentations of symptoms to obtain stimulants for abuse or diversion. Assessments in these cases consume valuable psychiatry time. In addition, some inmates apply intense pressure (i.e., coercion or extortion) to obtain controlled substances from peers receiving appropriately prescribed stimulant medications. Custody personnel must remain alert to deliberate misuse of these medications and to coerced diversion. Special handling and documentation of controlled substances also consume nursing time. Thus, the assessment and management of ADHD symptoms can increase workloads for clinical and custody staff.

ADHD, however, is a psychiatric condition that can significantly impair an inmate's functioning. Inattention to directives, poor planning with diminished consideration of consequences, poor frustration tolerance, and impulsivity can lead to dysfunction, disruptive behavior, and disciplinary infractions. ADHD diminishes an inmate's ability to participate in work, education, and programming. Despite the effect on staff workload, clinicians should consider ADHD in the differential diagnosis of an inmate's presentation, apply efforts to confirm or exclude it, and treat it when necessary to improve inmate functioning and diminish facility disruption.

Treatment modalities for ADHD include psychoeducation, cognitive-behavioral therapies, and controlled and noncontrolled medications. Therapy-based interventions can assist with the inmate's adaptation to the challenges of the correctional environment while having symptoms of inattention. The effectiveness of stimulants in reducing the symptoms of ADHD is well established. A ban on stimulants deprives inmates with legitimate needs of access to effective treatment.

Inmates with significant impairment in current participation in work, education, programming, or other meaningful activities due to ADHD should receive appropriate treatment. This includes access to stimulant medications if other interventions, including nonstimulant medications, are contraindicated or insufficient to adequately improve functioning. Evidence of active misuse of substances in the correctional setting, however, contraindicates prescription of stimulants. Whenever possible, observations from correctional officers, work supervisors, programming staff, teachers, and others can help confirm the presence of current functional impairment and response to treatment.

A recommended approach (Appelbaum 2009) to deciding which inmates to treat for ADHD begins with a review of current activities and functioning. Because of the challenges and risks associated with prescribing controlled substances, only those inmates actively engaged in, or attempting to engage in, productive work, education, and programming would have potential eligibility for treatment with stimulant medications. Difficulty in leisure activities alone, for example, would not meet this criterion. In addition, treatment based solely on disruptive behavior due to ADHD runs the risk of encouraging harmful acts by inmates seeking stimulants. Accordingly, inmates who have, or seek, no involvement in meaningful activities need no further workup for stimulant treatment.

In contrast, those inmates who have persistent inattention and/or hyperactivity or impulsivity that interferes with current productive functioning do warrant further assessment. The assessment typically includes obtaining observations by third parties (e.g., correctional officers, work supervisors, teachers) and a review of childhood information and records if available. As resources permit, use of observer and self-report rating scales and neuropsychological testing can help identify functional deficits and aid with diagnosis and monitoring. During the clinical examination, the psychiatrist also must assess for comorbidity and alternative symptom etiology.

When pharmacological intervention is supported by the complete evaluation, the psychiatrist may begin treatment with nonstimulant medications unless contraindicated or unsuccessful for the inmate. If stimulants prove necessary, use of shorter-acting and crushable agents can lessen the risk of diversion. Some of these considerations may involve off-label, but evidence-based, pharmacotherapy. The psychiatrist should usually make continued prescription of stimulant medications contingent on the inmate's engagement in any recommended nonpharmacological interventions for ADHD (e.g., education and therapy) and absence of current use of illicit substances.

A systematic approach to assessment and decision making can lessen unwarranted administrative and clinical burdens and reduce the risk of medication misuse while still ensuring that inmates with legitimate needs receive treatment.

Treatment Issues: Specific Populations

Women

The number of incarcerated women is rising at a rate that exceeds the rate for men. Although men still comprise the overwhelming majority of incarcerated individuals, access to medical and mental health care is equally important for women. Historically, psychiatric and other treatment programs for women have been based on treatment models designed for men. Studies show that the rates of SMI for women entering a jail or prison setting are significantly higher than for women in the community and are greater than the rates for incarcerated men (Fazel and Danesh 2002; Steadman et al. 2009). Rates of major mood and psychotic disorders are high, and PTSD is particularly prevalent (Trestman et al. 2007).

Female inmates frequently encounter different stressors before, during, and after incarceration than their male counterparts. Most women in correctional settings are mothers and have at least one child for whom they have been the primary caregiver prior to incarceration. Women who are pregnant during their incarceration are especially vulnerable. More than 75% of women entering correctional settings report a history of emotional, physical, or sexual abuse as a child or adult (Moloney et al. 2009). They have higher rates of domestic violence victimization than men. Incarcerated women have greater risk than men for sexually transmitted diseases and HIV because of prostitution, higher rates of substance use disorders, and drug offense arrests and are more likely to be victims of sexual assault while incarcerated.

Women, in general and in correctional settings, have a higher degree of treatment engagement in mental health services than men. Clinical staffing ratios have to reflect the relevant needs, including consideration of gender-specific stressors described here and willingness to participate in services. For example, facilities need to provide comprehensive postpartum mental health evaluations to minimize the risk of postpartum depression and psychosis; education for all staff and inmates about what constitutes sexual harassment and abuse; and access to adequate psychotherapeutic modalities, including cognitive-behavioral and group interventions.

Clinical and custody staff require training in gender-specific issues when working with female inmates. This training helps staff to recognize different symptom presentations, respond to different coping styles, provide appropriate treatment, and be sensitive to histories of abuse and trauma, especially when considering the use of forced medication or seclusion and restraints. Male inmates face many of the same challenges, and these principles may also apply to them.

Youth in Adult Correctional Facilities

For the purposes of these guidelines, a *youth* is defined as an inmate younger than age 18 years. The United States still tries some juveniles in adult criminal courts. At the time of this writing, New York and North Carolina automatically charge individuals 16 years of age and older as adults; 10 other states plus the District of Columbia automatically charge individuals 17 years of age and older as adults. In many states, certain felony offenses committed by adolescents are moved to adult criminal court. This practice has led to an increase in the detention and incarceration of younger offenders in adult jails and prisons. Data reflect rates of SMI among incarcerated adolescents that are substantially above those found in the community (Fazel et al. 2008).

Although there are limited systematic data on the number and ages of youth in adult correctional facilities, there appears to be an increasing national trend toward incarcerating younger individuals. Recent scientific inquiry and legal recognition has focused on differences between adolescents and adults, especially in brain development. This emerging literature on adolescents has revealed developmental immaturity, increased risk taking, testing of rules and limit setting, behavioral dyscontrol, and heightened desire for peer group affiliation and validation (all of which may pose challenges to staff, administrators, and clinicians within correctional settings).

Youth have a wide range of chronological and developmental maturity. This has clinical implications complicated by differences in 1) seriousness of offense; 2) stage of court proceeding and legal status (whether the juvenile will be tried in juvenile/family court or waived/transferred to adult criminal court); 3) legal history (e.g., first-time offender versus repeat offender, multiple incarcerations); 4) gang affiliation; 5) family and psychosocial resources or other supports; 6) youth and family's attitudes toward law enforcement, the court, state social services, or medical and mental health services; and 7) diversity issues such as race, culture, ethnicity, religion, sexual activity, and gender identity (Penn and Thomas 2005).

The presence of young inmates, who may be physically and emotionally immature, has led to a plethora of challenges for correctional systems. Youth with mental disorders present a special challenge. Only juveniles charged with the most serious crimes or with the most extensive and violent criminal histories are typically transferred to an adult court. As a group, they are likely to be especially impulsive, treatment resistant, and potentially violent. The presence of these youthful offenders in adult settings causes important and challenging problems for correctional administrators and custody and clinical staff (Penn and Thomas 2005). These problems include the likelihood that these youth have engaged in a pattern of high-risk-taking activities, substance abuse, school truancy, and other delinquent behaviors. Many have histories of physical and sexual victimization and exposure to traumatic events. There is the real possibility of revictimization either by adults or by fellow minors.

Because of their developmental immaturity and impulsivity, youthful offenders often engage in oppositional and defiant behaviors. Some observers have reported high levels of psychopathology, learning disorders, low intelligence, other developmental delays, fetal alcohol effects, neurological impairment, and disruptive behavior disorders such as ADHD, oppositional defiant disorder, and conduct disorder among young inmates. While housed in jail settings awaiting their legal disposition and possible waiver or transfer to the adult system, many adolescents face great anxiety based on the uncertainties of their cases and terrifying myths or fantasies about the jail or prison experience. Convicted felons whose sentences represent a relatively higher percentage of their lives (e.g., a 16-year sentence feels like "life" in prison to a 16-year-old boy) may perceive themselves as having "little to lose," which increases their risk of self-harm, attempted or completed suicide, impulsivity, behavioral dyscontrol, and dangerousness within the facility.

The Juvenile Justice and Delinquency Prevention Act (JJDPA; Pub. L. No. 93-415, 42 U.S.C. § 5601 et seq. [1974]) outlines requirements for juveniles in the criminal justice system. The JJDPA is currently the primary federal law intended to protect such youth. The JJDPA has four core requirements for state systems: deinstitutionalization of status offenders, separation of juveniles from adults in secure facilities, removal of juveniles from adult jails and lockups, and reduction of disproportionate minority contact in the juvenile justice system.

Because of the JJDPA, the Prison Rape Elimination Act, and the risk of state and federal litigation, most correctional systems have attempted to increase the safety of minors in adult correctional settings through sight and sound separation from adult prisoners. This response, however, may create barriers to educational, recreational, and treatment programming; limits contact exclusively to other youth who are equally immature, impulsive, and potentially violent; risks isolation when the peer group is very small; and precludes contact with more mature incarcerated adults who might model adaptive and prosocial prison behaviors. In contrast, youth with unsupervised access to older inmates have a greater risk of exploitation or of a strengthening of their identification with a criminal lifestyle.

Justice-involved youth have a high prevalence of risk factors for suicide (Hayes 2004; National Commission on Correctional Health Care 2007). Many young prisoners have experienced severe physical, sexual, and emotional abuse and neglect leading to trauma-related anxiety and depressive disorders, especially PTSD, that require mental health intervention. Some confined youth engage in self-injurious behavior and suicide attempts, and facilities need comprehensive suicide prevention policies and programming that reduce this risk.

Screening is no less important for youth than for adults. It is expected that each youth will require some mental health evaluation and referral, even when there is no identifiable history of mental health or medication treatment. Adult correctional systems that house youth typically require mental health evaluation of every minor. The evaluation should include special attention to intelligence, history of mental health treatment, special educational needs, and histories of emotional disturbances that often may have gone undetected.

Ideally, adult correctional facilities housing youthful offenders should have access to mental health professionals with experience in working with adolescents. At the very least, staff who work with these youth need additional or specialized training in identification of emerging emotional problems and when and how to refer youth for additional mental health and psychiatric treatment. They also will need special orientation to community services, if any, that will be available to the youth on release.

Incarceration of juveniles in adult settings, however tragic, presents some opportunities. For example, conditions nearly untreatable in an adult may be treatable in a teenager. Many youth with learning disabilities, or those struggling with school truancy or expulsion, have severe educational deficits that can be remedied in this setting. Furthermore, legal mandates for educational programming for adolescents actually may increase the resources available for this population.

When evaluating incarcerated youth, psychiatrists need to use a biopsychosocial model with attention to unique adolescent developmental, peer, gender, cultural, religious, and family issues. The assessment includes history of trauma, peer and family relationships and functioning, and family psychopathology (domestic violence, physical and sexual abuse, family criminality, substance abuse, or mental illness). A detailed assessment of the youth's past exposure to violence and perpetration of violent or illegal behaviors is essential. Psychiatrists should also carefully elicit any history of high-risk behaviors—unprotected intercourse, promiscuity, multiple partners, gang activities, prostitution, running away—and comorbid eating disorders, somatoform disorders, and gender dysphoria.

Psychiatrists often evaluate youthful offenders presenting with insomnia, depression, disruptive behaviors, or other symptoms. Many youth in the juvenile justice and adult correctional system are on multiple medications when initially detained, but others have never received medications; a comprehensive psychiatric assessment, when clinically indicated, provides an opportunity to reassess their treatment needs.

Psychotropic medication use requires caution and review of the potential risks, benefits, side effects, and alternatives with the youth and the youth's parent or legal guardian if the youth is still a minor. State mental health codes usually require a signed informed consent for minors. Use of multiple psychotropic medications—polypharmacy—requires caution because of potential risks, medication interactions, and side effects. Newly detained youth on psychiatric medications need careful assessment and monitoring, including serial reevaluations or gradual reductions in the number of medications while the youth is housed in a contained, structured, and supervised setting. Ideally, to ensure that the treatment trial proceeds safely and under supervision, medication changes follow clarification or resolution of a youth's legal disposition and placement.

Informed consent poses challenges because many youth have limited legal ability to consent to treatment and have "burned bridges" with their families of origin by the time they reach adult corrections. Special attention must be paid to gaining legally adequate informed consent, often through the use of treatment guardians. Similarly, clinicians may have conflicting duties to inform parents about the youth's care and, concomitantly, to maintain the youth's confidentiality.

With or without family involvement, these young prisoners are likely to have intense psychological and social work needs relating to their families of origin. These needs may include confronting intense anger over past neglect, abuse, and inconsistent or unavailable parenting; negotiating better relationships in the future, especially regarding family visitation; helping with problem solving for the receipt of bad news; identification and management of disappointment and frustration regarding canceled or no-show visits, family inconsistency, and lack of support; and preparation when release to the community is imminent.

Because of their involvement in the juvenile and adult justice systems, many of these high-risk youth may not have had the opportunity to experience normal developmental and maturational steps. Interestingly, many desire structure, rules, reliable adult role figures, and a predictable daily schedule. They may do very well with clear and consistent rules and with behavioral incentives.

Clinicians should recognize that while all seek the "best interests" of an incarcerated juvenile, a dynamic tension exists between the safety, security, and punishment approach of custody staff and the rehabilitative or therapeutic approach of clinicians. Each of the institutional service areas has its own legal mandates. Thus, it is paramount to learn the strengths, weaknesses, communication patterns, and relationships among mental health clinicians, direct care and other professional staff, outside agencies that interface with or provide other services to the juvenile correctional facility, educational staff and systems, and local medical staff (e.g., nursing, pediatric, dental).

The formulary, too, has to reflect the needs of these younger patients. Pharmacy and therapeutic committees and leaders who make decisions about formulary medications need to review the risks and benefits of medications that are typically restricted in adult correctional settings (e.g., psychostimulants, α_2-adrenergic agents, newer mood stabilizer and antidepressant agents, atypical antipsychotics) and the likelihood of polypharmacy and off-label medication treatment of youth in the community.

Special challenges often arise when youth approach community release. Because they may never have been able to "make it on the street," or because of intense familial conflict or unavailability, gang conflicts, or other psychosocial stressors, many youth offenders become extremely anxious, and even self-destructive, as their release date nears. Some will commit obvious and easily detectable infractions in order to forestall release. Mental health clinicians may be crucial in easing this transition through psychotherapy and referral to support services in the community.

Geriatric Persons

Effective access to mental health services for older inmates requires recognition of the special challenges facing inmates and mental health professionals, especially as the number of offenders older than age 65 in state and federal prisons increased at 94 times the rate of the overall sentenced population between 2007 and 2010 (Fellner 2012). The dramatic increase in the number of elderly inmates in correctional facilities over the past decade represents a humanitarian crisis. The causes include increasing life expectancy, harsher sentencing practices (long sentences, including life without parole), and, paradoxically, better health care in correctional facilities.

The National Institute of Corrections suggests that it may be useful to consider inmates older than age 50 as more likely to have common problems of aging even though the standard in the community is usually age 65. This relatively young definition for the geriatric inmate population is supported by the relatively high "biological age" of inmates due to substance abuse, poor nutrition, lack of prior medical care, lower socioeconomic status in the community, and other factors.

Older inmates have special medical needs that sometimes present with psychiatric symptoms or sequelae and affect psychiatric intervention, medications, relevance of counseling, structure of programming time, and housing. The problems are often chronic, persistent, progressive, related to the possibility of dying in custody, and expensive. Older inmates may also have environmental needs such as cells retrofitted with grab bars, handicap toilets, and facilities that accommodate wheelchairs.

Special psychosocial concerns that older inmates face may include

- Lack of connection to other inmates in the general population
- Physical vulnerability to serious consequences of assault
- Difficult and prolonged adjustment to a new environment
- Higher rate of suicide
- Greater likelihood of dying during incarceration
- Higher incidence of loss of external supports (e.g., spouse, parents, and friends)

Isolation may exacerbate or create mental illness or psychiatric crisis for older inmates. Some of them may benefit from mental health intervention, including group or peer counseling.

Clinical staff need training and competence in the special needs and care required by older inmates, and they can help educate custody staff to recognize and deal with cognitively impaired inmates who might not respond appropriately to a direct order.

Lesbian, Gay, Bisexual, and Transgender Persons

Trauma and stigma experienced by lesbian, gay, bisexual, or transgender (LGBT) individuals can increase their psychological distress and decrease their willingness to seek mental health services. When incarcerated, they risk additional discrimination and abuse. Compared with heterosexual inmates, studies have reported that they have 10 times the rate of sexual victimization by other inmates and up to 3 times the rate of sexual victimization by staff (Beck et al. 2013). This risk needs consideration on arrival at any correctional facility.

LGBT individuals differ in degree of comfort with their sexual orientation or gender identity and whether they are "out" or "closeted." Their choice about disclosure can change when moving from the community to jail or prison and between institutions. A respectful and nonjudgmental approach by the correctional psychiatrist can help LGBT inmates explore their choices and cope with their concerns. Transgender inmates, for example, may feel distress when housed in settings that do not allow them to express their gender identity or when they elect to stay closeted because of safety concerns. A therapeutic relationship in which they feel known by someone safe can improve emotional well-being.

Differences in issues and experiences exist among and within LGBT groups. For example, lesbians may encounter sexism, gay men have especially high rates of sexually transmitted infections and illicit drug use, and bisexuals sometimes find incomplete acceptance within either LGBT or heterosexual communities. In contrast to sexual orientation terminology (*lesbian, gay,* and *bisexual*), *transgender* refers to individuals who experience themselves differently from their natal gender. They may express a preference to be addressed by a name and a gender-defining pronoun that represents their desired gender. They may also want interventions such as hormones or sex reassignment surgery.

When assessing LGBT inmates, psychiatrists should avoid assumptions about how their patients view their sexual orientation or gender identity. Individuals vary widely in their experience of these issues, their degree of comfort and self-acceptance, and their mental health needs. Some use drugs to allay anxiety, improve self-comfort, or enhance sexuality, and a sensitive inquiry about drug use can convey knowledge and concern about their feelings. Although homophobia and discrimination may exacerbate symptoms of anxiety or depression, LGBT individuals should receive standard treatments for psychiatric disorders when present. Individuals who begin to accept and express repressed sexual orientation or gender identity may have emotional lability and heightened sexuality that can mimic a manic state.

Correctional facilities need to assess and address the safety needs of LGBT inmates. Housing units based solely on sexual orientation or gender identity, however, can lead to labeling and demoralization and do not substitute for other protective interventions. Isolation or segregation for safety may be appropriate only as an urgent and interim measure pending other safeguards.

Correctional systems do not have uniform policies about permissible treatment for transgender inmates. They differ on whether they allow access to gender-preferred clothing and toiletries or continuation or initiation of hormones. None have provided sex reassignment surgery, but this may change in response to ongoing litigation by transgender inmates. Consistent with the prevailing position of professional medical organizations, including the American Psychiatric Association (APA), courts and society in general are increasingly recognizing gender dysphoria as a medical condition appropriate for treatment.

Correctional psychiatrists can help foster awareness among custody and medical colleagues of the challenges faced by LGBT inmates, their mental health needs, and prevailing standards for their care.

Veterans

Another population that warrants focused attention is military veterans. The term *veteran* can have different meaning for different individuals, and correctional facilities need to screen individuals for a history of military service. The experience of veterans can vary significantly, ranging from no deployment to multiple tours of duty and combat exposure, especially for individuals who have served in recent military conflicts such as Operation Iraqi Freedom (Iraq) and Operation Enduring Freedom (Afghanistan). According to a Bureau of Justice Statistics report, 10% of prisoners in 2004 reported prior service in the U.S. Armed Forces (Noonan and Mumola 2007). Most of these individuals had served during wartime, and a quarter had seen combat duty. Almost all who reported military service were male inmates. Crimes included violent, nonviolent, and sexual offenses.

Many studies have highlighted the "invisible wounds of war" that include mental illness, substance use, PTSD, and traumatic brain injury. Each of these disorders may affect behavior and functioning and can go unrecognized without appropriate screening. Incarcerated veterans also have a heightened risk for suicide. Irritability, hypervigilance, and disinhibition from traumatic brain injuries can increase the risk of physical aggression. Clinical assessment can help in determining the appropriateness of disciplinary action in correctional environments.

Correctional facilities need mechanisms for identifying individuals who have a history of military service. Self-reports may be inaccurate. Some individuals do not want their military history known because of shame or potential loss of benefits for themselves or their families, and others may misunderstand the wording in screening questions about military status. For example, some persons who do not receive Veterans Administration (VA) benefits or had not faced combat or deployment may not consider themselves veterans and would answer "no" to the question of whether they are veterans. Some correctional facilities work with the VA or other government entities to try to identify these individuals through a data match.

Veteran status is important to identify for programming within the institution and for reentry planning. Careful assessment of military experience helps with treatment selection. Studies examining justice-involved veterans have begun to identify a significant portion with premilitary trauma in addition to trauma from their military experience. Military sexual trauma is increasingly recognized as an important factor that can influence the development of adjustment difficulties. Although originally identified as an issue for females in the military, it has also emerged as a critical issue for males who have served in the military. Individuals with a history of military sexual trauma may be particularly vulnerable to further sexual trauma in correctional environments. Facilities need trauma-informed services that recognize the unique aspects of military trauma.

Military history and veteran status have important reentry implications for veteran-focused community supports and benefits. Service members, veterans, and their families may each be affected by an individual's readjustment to civilian life. Furthermore, incarceration may reduce crucial financial supports available to immediate family members. Thus, reentry planning should include inquiry into benefits and potential entitlements. Individuals who were not honorably discharged may have reduced or no military benefits. In some cases, the military discharge status may have resulted from mental illness or substance use disorders and may be revisited. Inmates can get a copy of their DD 214 from the National Archives of Military Service to examine their military records and records of separation. Appeals of negative separations may be made.

Some programs allow for diversion and reentry supports for justice-involved veterans. For example, the VA Health Care for Re-entry Veterans (HCRV) Program assists incarcerated veterans with community reentry planning and provides linkages to treatment services, employment, housing, short-term case management, and other supports. Reentry coordinators in correctional facilities need to know about such programs.

Persons With Intellectual and Developmental Disabilities

Offenders with co-occurring mental illness and intellectual or developmental disability encounter unique difficulties in the criminal justice system and have special treatment needs (Hayes et al. 2007).

Intellectual disability involves significantly subaverage intellectual functioning and impairments in adaptive functioning with onset prior to age 18. Individuals with intellectual disability have diagnosable psychiatric disorders at rates three to four times greater than the general population (American Psychiatric Association 2013a, p. 40). Estimates vary widely because of the inherent difficulty in assessing behavioral manifestations of symptoms in persons with deficits in receptive and expressive language skills. Self-injurious behavior may occur because of a depressive disorder, diminished ability to tolerate stress, anxiety, impulsivity, or a learned behavior to increase attention from others. Deficits in communication skills contribute to the difficulty in assessing the patient. Often, medications are prescribed to target behavioral manifestations or symptoms instead of an underlying psychiatric disorder.

Inmates with intellectual or developmental disability and co-occurring mental disorders are unfortunately the most likely to be preyed on and ridiculed by other inmates. Their inability to process information rapidly or to comprehend instructions, their low frustration tolerance, and their impulsivity may have severe disciplinary consequences. Custody and treatment staff need additional training and education on intellectual and developmental disabilities to lessen the likelihood that they misperceive behaviors as intentional rule infractions or attribute them solely to intellectual disability while an SMI goes untreated. In addition, administrative, treatment, and custody staff need to know that the Americans with Disabilities Act (104 Stat. 330, 42 U.S.C. §§ 12111–12117 [1990]) applies to this population and requires "reasonable accommodation" for their needs.

Screening must include assessment of intellectual and adaptive functioning, review of participation in special education programs in school, and history of head injury and seizure disorder. Facility staff or outside consultants may need to further evaluate the nature and severity of limitations, administer individual intelligence tests, assess daily living skills, and obtain educational records or disability agency service records.

Each inmate's needs must be assessed individually. An inmate with intellectual or developmental disability may be capable of, or even prefer, being housed in the general population with minimal support because of the limited choices available to inmates and the predictability of inmate schedules. Others, however, require additional support, protection, or scrutiny by mental health and custody staff. Such support may involve employing a specialized correctional case worker with additional training or expertise and a smaller caseload or placing the offender in specialized housing or programs, including continuing special education programs. Depending on the size of the population, correctional facilities or systems may develop designated housing units for inmate protection, but they must ensure that offenders with intellectual or developmental disability and mental illness receive and participate in services or programs available to other inmates.

Hospice

A *terminal illness* is defined as an illness that, despite treatment, will likely result in death within a year. Dying with dignity and in compassionate surroundings may be more difficult to achieve in custody than in community settings. Caring for inmates with terminal illnesses may involve a defined hospice, either inside the prison (less likely to be needed in jail) or in an external contract facility, or consideration of compassionate release. Training and written policies need to address use of these options where available.

For larger correctional systems, a hospice that provides palliative care may be more useful for housing individuals who have a likelihood of dying while in custody from an identifiable illness (Yampolskaya and Winston 2003). The hospice patient may become more incapacitated and less oriented and behave more inappropriately as the disease and deterioration progress. Use of inmate volunteers (hospice workers) who are trained in basic health issues, universal precautions, and mobility management (Hoffmann and Dickinson 2011) may provide valuable assistance and reduce the dying patient's (or his or her family's) perception that "the prison isn't doing enough." Group therapy, end-of-life planning, and suicide prevention are interventions that psychiatrists can provide directly or assist other mental health professionals to provide.

Compassionate release in some cases may have advantages, including potential cost savings for the prison health care system and opportunities for patients and families to achieve closure. Perception of problems with public safety may decrease the viability of this option for individual patients.

Professional organizations, including the APA, can advise policymakers on reforms that assure up-to-date, evidence-based, and humane care for this population.

Mental Illness and Segregation

The widespread use of prolonged segregation in correctional systems in the United States creates unnecessary and avoidable risks to the health of individual inmates and to the public when those inmates return to the community. *Segregation* in this document refers to isolation of an inmate in a cell for an average of 23 hours per day with limited direct human interaction. The term *prolonged* as used here refers to stays in such settings exceeding 30 days. Under current practices, many inmates with an SMI spend months, years, or decades in segregation with little to no programming, which often results in substantial distress and harm.

Zinger and Wichmann (1999) provided a useful literature review on the psychological effects of 60 days in segregation. They pointed out that the early literature in this area is conflicting, filled with speculations, and often based on far-fetched extrapolations and generalizations. Methodological shortcomings apparent from reviewing more recent literature include reliance on anecdotal evidence, response bias, nonexistent or poor comparison groups, wide variation regarding the conditions of confinement in different prisons, cross-sectional instead of longitudinal design, and an overreliance on field and laboratory experiments pertinent to sensory deprivation (Gendreau and Labrecque, in press; Perrien and O'Keefe 2015). Mental health clinicians, however, frequently report that inmates without preexisting serious mental disorders can develop irritability, anxiety, and other dysphoric symptoms when housed in segregation units for long periods (Metzner 2002). Kaba et al. (2014) found at least one period of solitary confinement to have a significant association with self-harm.

Zubek et al. (1969) conceptualized segregation units as having three main characteristics: social isolation, sensory deprivation, and confinement. Each of these elements can vary significantly, as will the responses by different inmates to the segregation experience. In general, decreased and altered social interactions appear to cause more mental health problems than does sensory deprivation. In fact, many segregation units impose sensory overstimulation (e.g., inmates yelling for communication purposes or for other reasons). Radios and television sets, which may be available in these housing units, can decrease or eliminate sensory deprivation, although the severe disruption in normal social interactions remains a problem (Metzner 2002). When sanctions exclude access to even these minimal diversions, however, inmates in segregation can experience adverse psychological effects from unrelenting inactivity and boredom. Most segregation units also severely limit access to exercise, sunlight, and fresh air, which can have additional detrimental effects on mental and physical health.

Gendreau and Labrecque (in press) described the two dominant schools of thought regarding the impact of segregation housing on an inmate's mental health. One school equates the segregation environment with torture, because it is perceived to be psychologically very harmful to inmates (Haney 2012; Jackson 1983). Another school's position is that in prisons that meet basic standards of humane care, segregation results in only some inmates experiencing negative effects, and those are generally few (Clements et al. 2007; Gendreau and Goggin 2013). The severity of conditions and differences in individual resiliency can influence the degree of effect that segregation has on inmates.

There is a growing movement by health care staff and national organizations within the United States to exclude inmates from long-term segregation housing (New York Civil Liberties Union 2012). These efforts at exclusion have been much more successful for inmates with SMI. Clinicians generally agree that placement of inmates with SMIs in settings with extreme isolation (e.g., lack of congregate time out of cell and no access to reading materials, television, radio, educational programming, or work assignments) is contraindicated because many of these inmates' psychiatric conditions will clinically deteriorate or not improve (American Psychiatric Association 1997). In other words, many inmates with SMIs are harmed when placed in such settings because they lack access to adequate structured psychosocial programming or activities. In addition to potential litigation, this is the main reason that an increasing number of so-called supermax facilities have been excluding these inmates from long-term segregation housing, often by providing them with specialized mental health programming housing units (Haddad 1999; Metzner 1998; Metzner and Dvoskin 2006).

In addition to the potentially harmful effects on inmates themselves, excessive use of segregation can also compromise public health and safety. Almost all inmates eventually are released from jail or prison. When this occurs directly from segregation settings or after periods of incarceration that included significant time spent in segregation, those inmates may be poorly prepared for adjustment outside the institution. Exposure to extended periods of social isolation, limited or absent programming, and often ineffective or detrimental punishment in an attempt to modify behavior can lessen an inmate's readiness to function successfully in society.

The APA developed a position statement (American Psychiatric Association 2012) that included the following:

> Prolonged segregation of adult inmates with serious mental illness, with rare exceptions, should be avoided due to the potential for harm to such inmates. If an inmate with serious mental illness is placed in segregation, out-of-cell structured therapeutic activities (i.e., mental health/ psychiatric treatment) in appropriate programming space and adequate unstructured out-of-cell time should be permitted. Correctional mental health authorities should work closely with administrative custody staff to maximize access to clinically indicated programming and recreation for these individuals.

The Society of Correctional Physicians (2013) also published a similar position statement.

Improvement in the conditions of confinement of long-term segregation, however, should be extended to all inmates in segregation settings.

Critical barriers to access for clinically indicated mental health care, monitoring, and treatment often exist when an inmate is housed in a segregation environment. When an inmate is segregated—for any reason—from the general population, the correctional facility staff's responsibility to address serious mental health needs remains in effect. Indeed, because of the stressful nature of segregation housing, facilities should make special efforts to assess and address mental health treatment needs in these settings.

Mental health staff should routinely do regular rounds in all segregation housing units that impose isolation (e.g., supermax settings, disciplinary segregation) as an additional mental health screening procedure. These rounds help to identify inmates who have adverse reactions during their confinements in extreme isolation. Use of a mental health liaison model with the correctional and health care staffs, along with the rounds process, can facilitate the timely identification of inmates with acute symptoms of mental illness and the provision of appropriate clinical interventions.

Although important for screening and triage, mental health rounds at the cell front do not substitute for clinically indicated assessment or treatment sessions. Such clinical interventions should occur out of cell in a safe setting that allows for adequate sound privacy.

In sum, prolonged segregation exposes individuals to potential psychological, physiological, and medical risks. Those with SMI have special vulnerability to the adverse effects of social isolation. Psychiatrists should assist correctional systems with the development of evidence-based behavioral interventions that avoid the potential harm of social isolation.

The following principles address essential mental health services for inmates in segregation housing:

- No inmate should be placed in segregation housing solely because of symptoms of mental illness unless there is an immediate and serious danger for which there is no other reasonable temporary alternative (American Psychiatric Association 1997). Segregation in this context does not refer to medical or psychiatric seclusion, which should follow state mental health law and professional practice. Inmates with an SMI who are a high suicide risk or have active psychotic symptoms should not be placed in segregation housing. Instead, they should be transferred to an acute psychiatric setting for stabilization and treatment. If placed in segregation housing solely because of symptoms of a mental illness because there is no other reasonable alternative, the placement should be very short in duration, with adequate monitoring and treatment, until an appropriate clinical setting is available.
- When an inmate is placed in segregated housing for appropriate correctional reasons, the facility remains responsible for meeting all of the

serious medical and psychiatric needs of that inmate. Thus, such inmates must receive any mental health services that are deemed clinically indicated, their segregation status notwithstanding, including psychiatric and counseling services. For inmates who need ongoing intensive security, the facility must ensure that the conditions of confinement allow safe but meaningful social contact, interactions, and programming.

- Inmates in segregation who decompensate and experience a psychiatric crisis, including but not limited to acute psychosis and significant depression with suicidal ideation, should be removed from segregation and transferred to an acute psychiatric treatment setting (e.g., a hospital or an infirmary). If they are returned to segregation, it should be in a unit that provides adequate structured and unstructured activities as described below.

- When housed in segregation settings that provide clinically appropriate programming and psychiatric treatment, inmates who are known to have mental health needs (especially those with a known history of SMI) must be assessed at least weekly by a QMHP. Such assessment is intended to identify and appropriately respond to changing clinical needs of the inmate.

- If an inmate with SMI is placed in segregation, adequate unstructured out-of-cell time should be scheduled (at least 10 hours per week), as must adequate out-of-cell structured therapeutic activities (i.e., mental health/psychiatric treatment) (Metzner and Dvoskin 2006). Such treatment should be responsive to the level of care clinically required and occur in appropriate programming space, and correctional mental health authorities should work closely with administrative custody staff to maximize access to clinically indicated programming and recreation for these individuals.

- Institutions must provide for regular rounds by a QMHP in all segregation housing areas. During these rounds, each inmate, regardless of mental health history, should be visited briefly so that any emerging problem can be assessed. The clinician should also communicate with segregation security staff in order to identify any inmates showing signs of mental deterioration or psychological problems. Provision of adequate mental health services to inmates in segregation housing is a critical reflection of and a crucial component of a facility's overall quality of care.

- A policy and procedure should be developed and implemented in order to provide mental health input into the disciplinary process. The mental health assessment should identify any potential mitigating factors related to an inmate's mental illness that contributed to the alleged disciplinary infraction. Although treating clinicians may provide information about an inmate's symptoms and functioning at the time of the infraction, they should not conduct formal assessments or provide testimony on culpability for the infraction because doing so could compromise their clinical relationships with the inmate.

- Correctional systems need to develop alternatives to prolonged segregation for inmates. Further studies are needed to examine the efficacy of different behavioral programs and activities to help identify which inmates respond best to which interventions.

Seclusion and Restraint

The principles and guidelines in this report are intended to supplement the standards published by the NCCHC, which require implementation of health care–related seclusion or restraint in a manner consistent with current community practice (National Commission on Correctional Health Care 2014a, 2014b). Such community practice incorporates substantial efforts to train staff in de-escalation skills and in use of less-restrictive alternatives to restraint or seclusion. As an APA resource document has stated, little guidance exists on use of current community practice standards, especially regarding time frames or housing settings, for inmates in seclusion or restraint (see Appendix 6). Regulations established by the Centers for Medicare and Medicaid Services (2014) govern the use of restraints and seclusion in community hospitals.

The APA resource document includes the following statement:

> Since few correctional facilities are participants in the Medicare or Medicaid systems, the rules established by [the Centers for Medicare and Medicaid Services] concerning the use of restraint and seclusion had little impact on the use of seclusion or restraint for mental health care purposes in correctional systems. As a result, many correctional health care systems have not developed policies, procedures, or practices that are consistent with the current community practice. In addition, the frequent lack of meaningful external review or oversight in many correctional facilities regarding their mental health care practices has contributed to correctional facilities not keeping pace with prevailing community standards. When correctional health care systems use seclusion or restraint for health care purposes, they should be held to a similar standard of care as community health facilities, just as correctional facilities are not permitted to perform intrusive medical interventions unless they are done in a manner consistent with the community standard in appropriate health care settings. (Metzner et al. 2007)

Correctional policies, procedures, and practices need to address the following issues:

- **Location:** Specify where inmates are secluded or restrained for mental health purposes. We recommend that this occur on a health unit.
- **Property:** In the absence of rare clinical contraindications, inmates secluded or restrained for mental health purposes should have a mattress, blanket, and clothing.
- **Time frames:** Specify time frames for obtaining initial orders from appropriate licensed independent practitioners conducting initial face-to-face assessments by the ordering clinician, trained registered nurse, or physician assistant; duration of orders; frequency of nursing checks and range-of-motion exercises; and documentation intervals.

Other issues to address in policies and procedures include, but are not limited to, the following:

- Time frames for monitoring by health and custody staff should be established.
- Provisions should be made for regular documented review by a QMHP and a physician or independently licensed medical provider. (The former provides education and instruction to the inmate about the behavioral requirements for removal from seclusion or restraint. The latter reviews inmate health status, intake and output, and daily medication administration.)
- Inmates on clinical seclusion should be monitored at least every 8 hours with documented well-being checks by registered nursing staff.
- Custody or health staff should provide constant observation with 15-minute documented checks by nursing staff to monitor circulation, bathroom breaks, change in mental or health status, and intake of fluids and nourishment for inmates in restraints.
- Inmates should have at least underwear, and preferably full clothing.
- Restraints should be used as a last resort in managing acutely agitated or suicidal inmates.
- Secluded inmates should have access to structured therapeutic programming whenever possible without compromising the security and safety of the institution.

Since the publication of the APA resource document, the Centers for Medicare and Medicaid Services has revised the regulations in the 1999 Interim Rule (Centers for Medicare and Medicaid Services 2006; Substance Abuse and Mental Health Services Administration 2007; U.S. Department of Health and Human Services 1999). For purposes of this section, the most significant change was an expansion of the rule to include trained registered nurses or physician assistants among the clinicians allowed to perform the required 1-hour face-to-face evaluation (if followed by a timely consultation with an appropriate licensed independent professional). Consistent with this change, the APA resource document has been modified as follows:

> This resource document recommends that the initial face-to-face assessment by a licensed independent professional, *appropriately trained/credentialed registered nurse or physician assistant,* occurs within four hours of the actual seclusion or restraint. All physicians and other licensed independent professionals (LIPs) should be appropriately trained in the use of seclusion and restraint. *If the face-to-face initial assessment is not performed by a physician, consultation should be obtained by the examining clinician with a physician appropriately trained in the use of seclusion or restraints, within the same four-hour timeframe.*

Telepsychiatry

Telepsychiatry here refers to the use of live videoconferencing to provide psychiatric services in correctional settings. Telepsychiatry supplements on-site psychiatry services in many correctional settings. Many state medical boards endorse the use of telemedicine and have promulgated rules on the practice of telemedicine and telepsychiatry and grant limited telemedicine licenses. State legislatures have passed laws governing the use of telemedicine and reimbursement for these services. The American Telemedicine Association and several mental health professional groups have developed practice guidelines for telepsychiatry (American Telemedicine Association 2013).

Correctional settings lend themselves well to telepsychiatry use. Often these facilities are in rural communities where access to psychiatric services is limited or absent. Studies have shown that patients who receive psychiatric services via videoconferencing have had no negative consequences and quickly adapt to the technology. The patient and psychiatrist are talking to each other in real time as though they were in the room with each other. Also, not having to transport the inmate to an off-site psychiatrist's office enhances community safety by avoiding inmate transportation. Another use of telepsychiatry is observation of a patient during after-hours crises or for suspected medication side effects. Using remote visualization may avoid the costs associated with emergency transportation.

Psychiatrists and other mental health staff need selection criteria to ensure the appropriateness of patients for videoconference services. Patients who are acutely psychotic or paranoid may have difficulty being seen remotely and may be unable to give consent to participate in this treatment modality. Video quality has to allow the clinician to assess signs such as involuntary movements. An advantage to this technique is that the clinician can video record abnormal involuntary movement examinations to more accurately assess any progression in movement disorders.

Telepsychiatry sessions are scheduled like other sessions with mental health professionals. The equipment may be used for other purposes in the clinic, so scheduling should be coordinated. If the facility uses stationary videoconferencing equipment, placement near the medical or psychiatric clinic areas in an office that provides sound privacy facilitates clinical access. Few correctional systems have wireless services, and even if they do, the equipment may need to be plugged into a hardwired Internet connection.

Institutions need policies and procedures on the use of telepsychiatry, and physicians have to understand the state laws and medical board rules governing the practice where patients reside. No federal guidelines exist on telepsychiatry. The general rule for community and nonfederal correctional settings is that psychiatrists may physically be in another state but must hold a license in the state in which the patients reside (American Telemedicine Association 2013).

It is preferable to see patients in a room in the clinic area in the presence of a professional, often a social worker or nurse, who knows the patient and is a member of the treatment team. Whenever possible, psychiatrists obtain medical records by fax, e-mail, or other means prior to the session, and patients provide documented consent to engage in telepsychiatry. At the end of the session, psychiatrists may complete and electronically submit forms, prescriptions, and orders as though they were at the site. In facilities that use electronic health records, the telepsychiatrist needs remote records access for documentation and orders.

Video transmission needs encryption that meets Health Information Portability and Accountability Act (HIPAA) guidelines. This is usually accomplished with HIPAA-compliant software that ensures secure transmission and records the session.

Telepsychiatry is becoming a more accepted practice in correctional settings and in the community as the shortage of psychiatrists increases. Greater comfort by correctional mental health professionals with this technology increases accessibility of expeditious services for patients.

Spiritual Lives of Inmates

Early notions of the opportunity for spiritual development during incarceration include the rehabilitation movement, which considered imprisonment as a method of reformation based on a religious framework that equated criminal behavior with sin. In this view, prisons were seen as institutions for moral reform. In the United States during the late 1700s, a growing interest in shifting from a paradigm of strict punishment to one of moral reform led a group in Pennsylvania to design a facility that would, theoretically, instill a sense of penitence in each prisoner's conscience and consciousness. This method centered on the belief that reflection on criminal behavior in a forced monastic environment would lead to the development of penitence, and thus the term *penitentiary* was born. Although the penitentiary concept was initially appealing, was well received by the public, and served as the model for prison design and construction around the world, this method of reform through solitary confinement was ultimately abandoned at Eastern State Penitentiary in the 1930s.

Inmates draw on many resources to assist their adaptation to incarceration, such as family contact, peer support, work, education, and spiritual pursuits, including the practice of faith-based traditions. The spiritual experience is a process of personal transformation, which often occurs in relation to and is expressed within a religious tradition and practice. This transformation can provide a source of inner liberation that transcends the physical barriers of concrete and bars.

Spiritual endeavors and religious practice may be infused in an inmate's daily life. Although not a formal component of the diagnostic system, inmates' spiritual orientation and its place in their worldview are key components of the psychological and emotional constitution and a source for developing resiliency. Psychiatrists and other clinicians should routinely inquire about the importance of spirituality and religious practice when conducting clinical assessments and providing treatment to inmates. Awareness of and support for this potential source of strength and meaning is an important part of assisting in successful adaptation to the correctional environment.

Correctional chaplains are key sources of support for inmates' spiritual growth and religious practice. Chaplains are members of the employed or volunteer staff of correctional facilities and provide pastoral care to inmates and, in some cases, their families. Although chaplains represent their religious communities, pastoral care may be delivered to inmates of all faith traditions if requested. Pastoral care is the ministry of providing care and counseling to members of a congregation or to anyone in an institutional setting. Many correctional chaplains are licensed counselors and can provide formal counseling services. Commonly delivered services include pastoral counseling, grief counseling, and relationship counseling. As they plan treatments for their patients, secular mental health professionals and psychiatrists in particular should know that pastoral counseling is available and applicable across a spectrum of overt religiosity (Young and Griffith 1989).

Staff correctional chaplains often act as religious program managers in facilities and coordinate the activities of different faith groups and religious volunteers. In this capacity, they advise on and implement religious program policy, including approved religious articles, diets, and practices. In doing so, chaplains contribute to the coordinated operation of correctional facilities and are valuable members of the larger team. Chaplains and other staff (often volunteers) typically provide faith-based programming that addresses social, emotional, spiritual, recreational, or life skill issues from a faith/spiritual perspective. Mental health staff and psychiatrists should understand the benefits of such programs and make referrals for inmates' participation. Many religious services have demonstrable psychological benefits (Anderson and Young 1988; Griffith et al. 1986).

Frequently, the facility chaplain coordinates programs such as Alcoholics Anonymous and Narcotics Anonymous that potentially benefit all detainees and inmates. Chaplains are also likely to be qualified for and interested in such roles as co-therapists for group therapy. The other group leader might be a psychiatrist, psychologist, nurse, or social worker. Creative combinations for therapy can address problems that might otherwise be neglected. Finally, when turning attention to the world outside the correctional environment and designing reentry plans, psychiatrists need awareness of the skills, experience, and willingness for collaboration that exist among clergy in the community (Young et al. 2003).

References

American Academy of Psychiatry and the Law: Ethics Guidelines for Forensic Psychiatry. Bloomfield, CT, American Academy of Psychiatry and the Law, 2005. Available at: http://www.aapl.org/docs/pdf/ETHICSGDLNS.pdf. Accessed July 19, 2014.

American Correctional Health Services Association: Statement of Ethics, 1990. Available at: http://www.achsa.org/mission-ethics-statement/. Accessed July 19, 2014.

American Psychiatric Association: Psychiatric Services in Jails and Prisons (Task Force Report 29). Washington, DC, American Psychiatric Association, 1989

American Psychiatric Association: Practice guideline for the treatment of patients with schizophrenia. Am J Psychiatry 154(4 suppl):1–63, 1997

American Psychiatric Association: Position statement on segregation of prisoners with mental illness. Arlington, VA, American Psychiatric Association, 2012. Available at: http://www.psychiatry.org/File%20Library/Learn/Archives/Position-2012-Prisoners-Segregation.pdf. Accessed July 19, 2014.

American Psychiatric Association: Diagnostic and Statistical Manual of Mental Disorders, 5th Edition. Arlington, VA, American Psychiatric Association, 2013a

American Psychiatric Association: The Principles of Medical Ethics With Annotations Especially Applicable to Psychiatry, 2013 Edition. Arlington, VA, American Psychiatric Association, 2013b. Available at: http://www.psychiatry.org/File%20Library/Practice/Ethics%20Documents/principles2013–final.pdf. Accessed July 19, 2014.

American Telemedicine Association: Practice Guidelines for Video-Based Online Mental Health Services. Washington, DC, American Telemedicine Association, 2013. Available at: http://www.americantelemed.org/docs/default-source/standards/practice-guidelines-for-video-based-online-mental-health-services.pdf?sfvrsn=6. Accessed August 13, 2014.

Anderson RG, Young JL: The religious component of acute hospital treatment. Hosp Community Psychiatry 39(5):528–533, 1988 3378749

Anno BJ: Correctional Health Care: Guidelines for the Management of an Adequate Delivery System. Washington, DC, National Institute of Corrections, 2001

Appelbaum KL: Attention deficit hyperactivity disorder in prison: a treatment protocol. J Am Acad Psychiatry Law 37(1):45–49, 2009 19297632

Appelbaum KL, Hickey JM, Packer I: The role of correctional officers in multidisciplinary mental health care in prisons. Psychiatr Serv 52(10):1343–1347, 2001 11585950

Appelbaum KL, Savageau JA, Trestman RL, et al: A national survey of self-injurious behavior in American prisons. Psychiatr Serv 62(3):285–290, 2011 21363900

Baillargeon J, Binswanger IA, Penn JV, et al: Psychiatric disorders and repeat incarcerations: the revolving prison door. Am J Psychiatry 166(1):103–109, 2009 19047321

Baillargeon J, Penn JV, Knight K, et al: Risk of reincarceration among prisoners with co-occurring severe mental illness and substance use disorders. Adm Policy Ment Health 37(4):367–374, 2010 19847638

Beck AJ, Berzofsky M, Caspar R, et al: Sexual Victimization in Prisons and Jails Reported by Inmates, 2011–12 (May 2013, NCJ 241399). Washington, DC, U.S. Department of Justice, Bureau of Justice Statistics, 2013. Available at: http://www.bjs.gov/content/pub/pdf/svpjri1112.pdf. Accessed July 17, 2014.

Centers for Medicare and Medicaid Services: Medicare and Medicaid Programs: hospital conditions of participation: patients' rights: final rule. Fed Regist 71(236):71378–71428, 2006

Centers for Medicare and Medicaid Services: CMS Manual System Publ. 100-07 State Operations Provider Certification (42 C.F.R. Part 482.13[e] and [f]). Baltimore, MD, Centers for Medicare and Medicaid Services, 2014. Available at: http://www.cms.gov/regulations-and-guidance/guidance/transmittals/downloads/r37soma.pdf. Accessed August 10, 2014.

Clements CB, Althouse R, Ax RK, et al: Systematic issues and correctional outcomes: expanding the scope of correctional psychology. Crim Justice Behav 34(7):919–932, 2007

Cloyes KG, Wong B, Latimer S, et al: Time to prison return for offenders with serious mental illness released from prison: a survival analysis. Crim Justice Behav 37(2):175–187, 2010

Cohen F: Practical Guide to Correctional Mental Health and the Law. Kingston, NJ, Civic Research Institute, 2011

Crosby SS, Apovian CM, Grodin MA: Hunger strikes, force-feeding, and physicians' responsibilities. JAMA 298(5):563–566, 2007 17666678

Cunnington D: Non-benzodiazepine hypnotics: do they work for insomnia? BMJ 346:e8699, 2013 23284161

Daines MK: Hunger strikes in correctional facilities, in Correctional Psychiatry. Edited by Thienhaus OJ, Piasecki M. Kingston, NJ, Civic Research Institute Inc, 2007, pp 8-1–8-12

Diamond PM, Wang EW, Holzer CE 3rd, et al: The prevalence of mental illness in prison. Adm Policy Ment Health 29(1):21–40, 2001 11811770

Ditton PM: Special Report: Mental Health and Treatment of Inmates and Probationers. Washington, DC, U.S. Department of Justice, Bureau of Justice Statistics, 1999

Fazel S, Danesh J: Serious mental disorder in 23000 prisoners: a systematic review of 62 surveys. Lancet 359(9306):545–550, 2002 11867106

Fazel S, Doll H, Långström N: Mental disorders among adolescents in juvenile detention and correctional facilities: a systematic review and metaregression analysis of 25 surveys. J Am Acad Child Adolesc Psychiatry 47(9):1010–1019, 2008 18664994

Fellner J: Old Behind Bars: The Aging Prison Population in the United States. New York, Human Rights Watch, 2012. Available at: http://www.hrw.org/sites/default/files/reports/usprisons0112webwcover_0_0.pdf. Accessed July 17, 2014.

Gendreau P, Goggin C: Practicing psychology in correctional settings, in The Handbook of Forensic Psychology, 4th Edition. Edited by Weiner IB, Otto RK. Hoboken, NJ, Wiley, 2013, pp 759–794

Gendreau P, Labrecque RM: The effects of administrative segregation: a lesson in knowledge cumulation, in Oxford Handbook on Prisons and Imprisonment. Edited by Wooldredge J, Smith P. Oxford, UK, Oxford University Press, in press

Griffith EEH, Mahy GE, Young JL: Psychological benefits of Spiritual Baptist "mourning," II: an empirical assessment. Am J Psychiatry 143(2):226–229, 1986 3946661

Haddad J: Treatment for inmates with serious mental illness who require specialized placement but not psychiatric hospitalization. Correct Mental Health Rep 59(1):60–62, 1999

Haney C: Testimony of Professor Craig Haney to the Senate Judiciary Subcommittee on the Constitution, Civil Rights, and Human Rights Hearing on Solitary Confinement. June 19, 2012. Available at: http://www.judiciary.senate.gov/imo/media/doc/12-6-19HaneyTestimony.pdf. Accessed July 21, 2014

Hayes LM: Juvenile Suicide in Confinement: A National Survey (NCJ 206354). Washington, DC, U.S. Department of Justice, Office of Juvenile Justice and Delinquency Prevention, 2004. Available at: https://www.ncjrs.gov/pdffiles1/ojjdp/grants/206354.pdf. Accessed March 11, 2015.

Hayes LM: National Study of Jail Suicide: 20 Years Later. Washington, DC, U.S. Department of Justice, National Institute of Corrections, 2010

Hayes S, Shackell P, Mottram P, et al: The prevalence of intellectual disability in a major UK prison. British Journal of Learning Disabilities 35(3):162–167, 2007

Hoffmann HC, Dickinson GE: Characteristics of prison hospice programs in the United States. Am J Hosp Palliat Care 28(4):245–252, 2011 20834030

Jackson M: Prisoners of Isolation: Solitary Confinement in Canada. Toronto, ON, Canada, University of Toronto Press, 1983

Kaba F, Lewis A, Glowa-Kollisch S, et al: Solitary confinement and risk of self-harm among jail inmates. Am J Public Health 104(3):442–447, 2014 24521238

Karberg JC, James DJ: Bureau of Justice Statistics Special Report: Substance Dependence, Abuse, and Treatment of Jail Inmates, 2002 (NCJ 209588). Washington, DC, U.S. Department of Justice, Office of Justice Programs, 2005. Available at: http://www.bjs.gov/content/pub/pdf/sdatji02.pdf. Accessed August 12, 2014.

Keram EA: Hunger strikes, in Oxford Textbook of Correctional Psychiatry. Edited by Trestman RL, Appelbaum KL, Metzner JL. New York, Oxford University Press, 2015, pp 365–369

Kraus SS, Rabin LA: Sleep America: managing the crisis of adult chronic insomnia and associated conditions. J Affect Disord 138(3):192–212, 2012 21652083

Lazarus J: Letter on behalf of the American Medical Association to Defense Secretary Chuck Hagel. April 25, 2013. Available at: http://www.jhsph.edu/research/centers-and-institutes/center-for-public-health-and-human-rights/_pdf/AMA%20Hunger%20Strikes%20Letter.pdf. Accessed August 12, 2014.

McKee J, Penn JV, Koranek A: Psychoactive medication misadventuring in correctional health care. J Correct Health Care 20(3):249–260, 2014 24934843

Metzner JL, Tardiff K, Lion J, et al: Resource document on the use of restraint and seclusion in correctional mental health care. J Am Acad Psychiatry Law 35(4):417–425, 2007 18086731

Metzner JL: An introduction to correctional psychiatry: part III. J Am Acad Psychiatry Law 26(1):107–115, 1998 9554715

Metzner JL: Class action litigation in correctional psychiatry. J Am Acad Psychiatry Law 30(1):19–29; discussion 30–32, 2002 11931366

Metzner J, Dvoskin J: An overview of correctional psychiatry. Psychiatr Clin North Am 29(3):761–772, 2006 16904510

Mitchell MD, Gehrman P, Perlis M, et al: Comparative effectiveness of cognitive behavioral therapy for insomnia: a systematic review. BMC Fam Pract 13:40, 2012 22631616

Moloney KP, van den Bergh BJ, Moller LF: Women in prison: the central issues of gender characteristics and trauma history. Public Health 123(6):426–430, 2009 19493553

Morin CM, Benca R: Chronic insomnia. Lancet 379(9821):1129–1141, 2012 22265700

National Commission on Correctional Health Care: Position Statement: Prevention of Juvenile Suicide in Correctional Settings. Chicago, IL, National Commission on Correctional Health Care, 2007. Available at: http://www.ncchc.org/prevention-of-juvenile-suicide-in-correctional-settings. Accessed July 17, 2014.

National Commission on Correctional Health Care: Standards for Mental Health Services in Correctional Facilities. Chicago, IL, National Commission on Correctional Health Care, 2008

National Commission on Correctional Health Care: Standards for Health Services in Jails. Chicago, IL, National Commission on Correctional Health Care, 2014a

National Commission on Correctional Health Care: Standards for Health Services in Prisons. Chicago, IL, National Commission on Correctional Health Care, 2014b

New York Civil Liberties Union: Boxed In: The True Cost of Extreme Isolation in New York's Prisons. New York, New York Civil Liberties Union, 2012. Available at: http://www.nyclu.org/files/publications/nyclu_boxedin_FINAL.pdf. Accessed March 11, 2014.

Noonan M, Ginder S: Mortality in local jails and state prisons, 2000–2011: statistical tables, in Bureau of Justice Statistics: Statistical Tables. Washington, DC, U.S. Department of Justice, Office of Justice Programs, August 2013. Available at: http://www.bjs.gov/content/pub/pdf/mljsp0011.pdf. Accessed August 4, 2014.

Noonan M, Mumola CJ: Bureau of Justice Statistics Special Report: Veterans in State and Federal Prison, 2004. Washington, DC, U.S. Department of Justice, Office of Justice Programs, May 2007. Available at: http://www.bjs.gov/content/pub/pdf/vsfp04.pdf. Accessed July 17, 2014.

Penn JV, Thomas C: Practice parameter for the assessment and treatment of youth in juvenile detention and correctional facilities. J Am Acad Child Adolesc Psychiatry 44(10):1085–1098, 2005 16175113

Perrien M, O'Keefe M: Disciplinary infractions and restricted housing, in Oxford Textbook of Correctional Psychiatry. Edited by Trestman RL, Appelbaum KL, Metzner JL. New York, Oxford University Press, 2015, pp 71–75

Rold WJ: Thirty years after Estelle v. Gamble: a legal retrospective. J Correct Health Care 14(1):11–20, 2008

Society of Correctional Physicians: Restricted Housing of Mentally Ill Inmates–Position Statement. Chicago, IL, Society of Correctional Physicians, 2013. Available at: http://societyofcorrectionalphysicians.org/resources/position-statements/restricted-housing-of-mentally ill-inmates. Accessed December 23, 2013.

Spaulding AC, Kim AY, Harzke AJ, et al: Impact of new therapeutics for hepatitis C virus infection in incarcerated populations. Top Antivir Med 21(1):27–35, 2013 23596276

Steadman HJ, Osher FC, Robbins PC, et al: Prevalence of serious mental illness among jail inmates. Psychiatr Serv 60(6):761–765, 2009 19487344

Substance Abuse and Mental Health Services Administration: Seclusion and restraint: final rule on patients' rights. SAMHSA News 15(1), 2007. Available at: http://www.samhsa.gov/samhsa_news/VolumeXV_1/article5.htm. Accessed July 15, 2014.

Trestman RL, Ford J, Zhang W, et al: Current and lifetime psychiatric illness among inmates not identified as acutely mentally ill at intake in Connecticut's jails. J Am Acad Psychiatry Law 35(4):490–500, 2007 18086741

U.S. Department of Health and Human Services, Health Care Finance Administration: Medicare and Medicaid programs: conditions of participation: patients' rights. Interim final rule, 42 CFR 482. Fed Regist 64:36069–36089, 1999

U.S. Department of Health and Human Services: Additional protections pertaining to biomedical and behavioral research involving prisoners as subjects (subpart C), in Code of Federal Regulations: Title 45, Public Welfare; Department of Health and Human Services, Part 46, Protection Of Human Subjects, 2009. Available at: http://www.hhs.gov/ohrp/humansubjects/guidance/45cfr46.html#subpartc. Accessed August 12, 2014.

U.S. Department of Justice: National Standards to Prevent, Detect, and Respond to Prison Rape; Final Rule (28 CFR part 115). Federal Register 77(119):37105–37232, June 20, 2012. Available at: http://www.gpo.gov/fdsys/pkg/FR-2012-06-20/html/2012-12427.htm. Accessed March 17, 2015.

World Medical Association: World Medical Association Declaration on Hunger Strikers (Declaration of Malta). Ferney-Voltaire, France, World Medical Association, 2006. Available at: http://www.wma.net/en/30publications/10policies/h31/. Accessed August 12, 2014.

Yampolskaya S, Winston N: Hospice care in prison: general principles and outcomes. Am J Hosp Palliat Care 20(4):290–296, 2003 12911074

Young JL, Griffith EEH: The development and practice of pastoral counseling. Hosp Community Psychiatry 40(3):271–276, 1989 2917737

Young JL, Griffith EEH, Williams DR: The integral role of pastoral counseling by African-American clergy in community mental health. Psychiatr Serv 54(5):688–692, 2003 12719499

Zinger I, Wichmann C: The Psychological Effects of 60 Days in Administrative Segregation. Ottawa, ON, Correctional Service of Canada Research Branch, 1999. Available at: http://www.csc-scc.gc.ca/research/092/r85_e.pdf. Accessed July 19, 2014.

Zubek JP, Bayer L, Shephard JM: Relative effects of prolonged social isolation and confinement: behavioral and EEG changes. J Abnorm Psychol 74(5):625–631, 1969 5349408

APPENDIXES

Position Statements and Resource Document of the American Psychiatric Association

1. Position Statement on Access to Comprehensive Psychiatric Assessment and Integrated Treatment, June 2009
2. Position Statement on Use of the Concept of Recovery, July 2005
3. Position Statement on Adjudication of Youths as Adults in the Criminal Justice System, December 2005
4. Position Statement on Mentally Ill Prisoners on Death Row, December 2005
5. Position Statement on Use of Jails to Hold Persons Without Criminal Charges Who Are Awaiting Civil Psychiatric Hospital Beds, July 2007
6. Resource Document: The Use of Restraint and Seclusion in Correctional Mental Health Care, December 2006
7. Position Statement on Capital Punishment: Adoption of AMA Statements on Capital Punishment, July 2008
8. Position Statement on Atypical Antipsychotic Medications, September 2009
9. Position Statement on Access to Care for Transgender and Gender Variant Individuals, July 2012
10. Position Statement on Segregation of Prisoners With Mental Illness, December 2012

APPENDIX 1

APA Official Actions

Position Statement on Access to Comprehensive Psychiatric Assessment and Integrated Treatment

Approved by the Board of Trustees, September 2009

Approved by the Assembly, May 2009

"Policy documents are approved by the APA Assembly and Board of Trustees....These are...position statements that define APA official policy on specific subjects..."

– *APA Operations Manual*

For patients referred for the treatment of mental illness:

- Restricting access to assessment by a psychiatrist and integrated treatment is not cost-effective.
- Delegating treatment to various specialties is a medical, not a procedural administrative or business decision.
- There are some situations in which split treatment has advantages, many situations in which it is inadvisable, and no situation for which it should be mandated by a health plan.

Prepared by the APA Committee on Managed Care: Paul H. Wick, M.D., Chair; Robert C. Bransfield, M.D., Co-chair; Gregory G. Harris, M.D.; George D. Santos, M.D.; Jonathan L. Weker, M.D.; Barry K. Herman, M.D.; Alan A. Axelson, M.D.; Anthony L. Pelonero, M.D.; Nicolas Abid, M.D.; and Joel Johnson, M.D.

APA supports screening and referral protocols by which:

- Any patient who is referred for mental healthcare should be properly screened and be seen by a psychiatrist early enough for meaningful clinical input towards the patient's comprehensive psychiatric assessment and to ensure attention and coordination of medical care for associated medical needs.
- Treatment planning should be based on a comprehensive assessment using the biopsychosocial perspective.
- Patients in need of treatment should not be barred from receiving combined psychotherapy and medication management from psychiatrists who are available and willing to offer it.

This is a revision of the 2002 position statement.

APPENDIX 2

APA Official Actions

Position Statement on Use of the Concept of Recovery

Approved by the Board of Trustees, July 2005

Approved by the Assembly, May 2005

"Policy documents are approved by the APA Assembly and Board of Trustees....These are...position statements that define APA official policy on specific subjects..."

– APA Operations Manual

The American Psychiatric Association endorses and strongly affirms the application of the concept of recovery to the comprehensive care of chronically and persistently mentally ill adults, including the concept of resilience in seriously emotionally disturbed children. The concept of recovery emphasizes a person's capacity to have hope and lead a meaningful life, and suggests that treatment can be guided by attention to life goals and ambitions. It recognizes that patients often feel powerless or disenfranchised, that these feelings can interfere with initiation and maintenance of mental health and medical care, and that the best results come when patients feel that treatment decisions are made in ways that suit their cultural, spiritual, and personal ideals. It focuses on wellness and resilience and encourages patients to participate actively in their care, particularly by enabling them to help define the goals of psychopharmacologic and psychosocial treatments.

The concept of recovery has a long history in medicine and its principles are important in the management of all chronic disorders. The concept of recovery enriches and supports medical and rehabilitation models. By applying the concept of recovery as well as rehabilitation techniques and by encouraging other mental health professionals to adopt the concept of recovery, psychiatrists can enhance the care of all clinical populations served within the community based and other public sector mental health and behavioral health systems.

The concept of recovery values include maximization of 1) each patient's autonomy based on that patient's desires and capabilities, 2) patient's dignity and self-respect, 3) patient's acceptance and integration into full community life, and 4) resumption of normal development. The concept of recovery focuses on increasing the patient's ability to successfully cope with life's challenges, and to successfully manage their symptoms. The application of the concept of recovery requires a commitment to a broad range of necessary services and should not be used to justify a retraction of resources.

The concept of recovery is predicated on a partnership between psychiatrist, other practitioners, and patient in the construction and direction of all services aimed at maximizing hope and quality of life.

APPENDIX 3

APA Official Actions

Position Statement on Adjudication of Youths as Adults in the Criminal Justice System

Approved by the Board of Trustees, December 2005

Approved by the Assembly, November 2005

> "Policy documents are approved by the APA Assembly and Board of Trustees....These are...position statements that define APA official policy on specific subjects..."
>
> – *APA Operations Manual*

The ostensible goals of transfer, or waiver, to the criminal justice system include: (1) deterrence of youth from committing crimes, (2) reduction in recidivism among youth who are transferred, and (3) improvement of public safety. However, instead of accomplishing their intended goals, waivers have seriously disrupted the lives of youth, and their families, especially those from minority communities. The federal government, in concert with states, should review and develop a strategy to reform current transfer/ waiver practices. The general goals of such reform must be: to reduce the number of youth inappropriately transferred to the criminal justice system who could be better served by the juvenile justice system, to provide rehabilitation services that support the development of youth as valued members of society, and to ensure community safety. Reform should specifically include:

1. a moratorium on the expansion of eligibility criteria for transfer.
2. limiting transfer only to judicial discretion (or sole authority by judge).

3. an elimination of transfers for nonviolent offenders.
4. an elimination of transfer of first-time offenders.
5. the development of specialized facilities for transferred youth. Such facilities would include small living units that are secure and safe; programming that addresses the developmental, educational, health, mental health, religious, and other special needs of these youth; and
6. adequately staffed with qualified workers to ensure safety and specialized programming (Council of Juvenile Correctional Administrators 2005).

APA Official Actions

Position Statement on Mentally Ill Prisoners on Death Row

Approved by the Board of Trustees, December 2005

Approved by the Assembly, November 2005

> "Policy documents are approved by the APA Assembly and Board of Trustees....These are...position statements that define APA official policy on specific subjects..."
>
> – *APA Operations Manual*

(a) **Grounds for Precluding Execution.** A sentence of death should not be carried out if the prisoner has a mental disorder or disability that significantly impairs his or her capacity (i) to make a rational decision to forego or terminate post-conviction proceedings available to challenge the validity of the conviction or sentence; (ii) to understand or communicate pertinent information, or otherwise assist counsel, in relation to specific claims bearing on the validity of the conviction or sentence that cannot be fairly resolved without the prisoner's participation; or (iii) to understand the nature and purpose of the punishment, or to appreciate the reason for its imposition in the prisoner's own case. Procedures to be followed in each of these categories of cases are specified in (b) through (d) below.

(b) **Procedure in Cases Involving Prisoners Seeking to Forgo or Terminate Post-Conviction Proceedings.** If a court finds that a prisoner under sentence of death who wishes to forgo or terminate post-conviction proceedings has a mental disorder or disability that significantly impairs his or her capacity to make a rational decision, the court should permit a next friend acting on the prisoner's behalf to initiate or pursue available remedies to set aside the conviction or death sentence.

(c) Procedure in Cases Involving Prisoners Unable to Assist Counsel in Post-Conviction Proceedings. If a court finds at any time that a prisoner under sentence of death has a mental disorder or disability that significantly impairs his or her capacity to understand or communicate pertinent information, or otherwise to assist counsel, in connection with post-conviction proceedings, and that the prisoner's participation is necessary for a fair resolution of specific claims bearing on the validity of the conviction or death sentence, the court should suspend the proceedings. If the court finds that there is no significant likelihood of restoring the prisoner's capacity to participate in post-conviction proceedings in the foreseeable future, it should reduce the prisoner's sentence to a lesser punishment.

(d) Procedure in Cases Involving Prisoners Unable to Understand the Punishment or Its Purpose. If, after challenges to the validity of the conviction and death sentence have been exhausted and execution has been scheduled, a court finds that a prisoner has a mental disorder or disability that significantly impairs his or her capacity to understand the nature and purpose of the punishment, or to appreciate the reason for its imposition in the prisoner's own case, the sentence of death should be reduced to a lesser punishment.

APPENDIX 5

APA Official Actions

Position Statement on Use of Jails to Hold Persons Without Criminal Charges Who Are Awaiting Civil Psychiatric Hospital Beds

Approved by the Board of Trustees, July 2007

Approved by the Assembly, May 2007

> "Policy documents are approved by the APA Assembly and Board of Trustees.... These are... position statements that define APA official policy on specific subjects..."
>
> – *APA Operations Manual*

Access to appropriate levels of care is essential for persons with mental illness. Where no criminal conduct has been alleged, persons determined to be in need of civil psychiatric commitment for treatment of acute psychiatric symptoms should not be held in jails or other correctional facilities.

The APA encourages psychiatrists to continue to work with local, state, and federal agencies to provide adequate mental health services for civil committees.

APPENDIX 6

The Use of Restraint and Seclusion in Correctional Mental Health Care

Resource Document

Approved by the Joint Reference Committee, December 2006

> "The findings, opinions, and conclusions of this report do not necessarily represent the views of the officers, trustees, or all members of the American Psychiatric Association. Views expressed are those of the authors."
>
> – *APA Operations Manual*

This resource document discusses the use of seclusion or restraint for purposes of mental health intervention in jails and prisons, in contrast to its use for correctional purposes (i.e., specifically custody reasons).[1] The use of seclusion or restraint for mental health reasons is an emergency measure to prevent imminent harm to the patient or other persons when other means of control are not effective or appropriate.

This Resource Document was produced by a workgroup of the Council on Psychiatry and Law, and reviewed and approved by the Council in September 2006.

Members of the workgroup included Jeffrey L. Metzner, M.D; Kenneth Tardiff, M.D., M.P.H.; John Lion, M.D.; William H. Reid, M.D.; Patricia Ryan Recupero, M.D., J.D.; and Diane H. Schetky, M.D. Consultants of the workgroup included Bruce M. Edenfield, J.D.; Marlin Mattson, M.D.; and Jeffrey S. Janofsky, M.D.

It is clear that there is a national movement to reduce the use of seclusion or restraint in mental health treatment, which is facilitated by treatment programs that focus on a plan of care that minimizes the need for it (National Technical Assistance Center for State Mental Health Planning 2002). The importance of establishing a therapeutic culture to partner with the patient for safety rather than to control the patient for safety has been emphasized. Assessment and treatment planning measures should focus on patient-specific approaches to the prevention and management of behavioral emergencies. Patients should participate in the treatment planning process to ascertain successful crisis resolution measures that are based on the patient's psychiatric condition, prior experience with behavioral emergencies, and risk for future harm.

Several major mental health organizations joined together to produce a useful guide to reducing seclusion and restraint use, *Learning From Each Other: Success Stories and Ideas for Reducing Seclusion and Restraint* (American Psychiatric Association et al. 2003). The appendix to that document includes a set of sample forms and checklists covering core skills and knowledge for direct care staff, patient- reported therapeutic interventions, de-escalation tips, and information relevant to the use of seclusion and restraint. The National Association of State Mental Health Program Directors Council (2001) and the National Technical Assistance Center for State Mental Health Planning (Huckshorn 2006) have also produced very useful publications aimed at reducing the use of seclusion and restraint.

The efforts in recent years to minimize the use of seclusion and restraint of persons with mental illness have been a positive development.

---

[1]The use of seclusion or restraint for correctional purposes is generally driven by classification and disciplinary issues unique to the correctional setting. For example, an inmate's security classification may require the use of handcuffs and leg irons (i.e., restraints) during movement outside of the inmate's cell or housing unit. Restraints may also be used by custody staff to control an inmate's assaultive behavior that is not related to mental illness. With few exceptions, cell extractions (both calculated use of force and on an emergency basis) by custody staff are governed by custody policies and procedures even when they involve mentally ill inmates. However, there are generally special provisions in such policies and procedures when such a use of force involves the mentally ill inmate that usually includes attempted assessment/intervention by mental health staff prior to the use of force. Disciplinary segregation has many characteristics similar to seclusion such as confinement to a cell and restricted access to personal belongings. Custody guidelines for using these security measures are generally very different than those relevant to the use of seclusion or restraint for mental health purposes and will not be addressed in this document.

However, the nature of severe mental illness is such that seclusion and restraint cannot be eliminated as a necessary part of treatment and management. Therefore, it is crucial that there not be an expectation that seclusion and restraint be abolished in correctional mental health. Staff must feel that they are permitted to use seclusion and restraint when it is clinically necessary for the welfare and safety of the patient, other patients and the staff. If staff are made to feel that these procedures should never be used and that using them, no matter what the circumstances, indicates that staff have done something very wrong and have failed in their jobs, they will be inclined to avoid seclusion and restraint even when it was the best alternative for the situation. The unintended consequences may include unnecessary injuries to the patient, to other patients and to the staff. Once it becomes known that a treatment setting has become a dangerous place to work, retaining and recruiting good staff to work there becomes very difficult. Experience has shown that under such circumstances, the quality of the treatment environment deteriorates.

The Need for This Resource Document

The second edition of a Task Force Report of the American Psychiatric Association (2000) entitled "Psychiatric Services in Jails and Prisons" reiterates that principles and guidelines in the Task Force's publication are intended to supplement the standards published by the National Commission on Correctional Health Care (2003a, 2003b). These standards essentially state that seclusion or restraint, when used for health care purposes, is implemented in a manner consistent with the current community practice. However, little guidance is provided regarding current community practices, especially in terms of relevant timeframes or settings where inmates in seclusion or restraint should be housed.

Community practices pertinent to the use of seclusion or restraint for mental health purposes may vary across jurisdictions because of differing rules and regulations promulgated by the state Department of Mental Health or equivalent agency. Relevant rules and regulations were significantly impacted and revised during July 1999, after the Health Care Financing Administration (HCFA), now called the Centers for Medicare and Medicaid Services (CMS), defined rules for the use of seclusion and restraint in facilities that participate in Medicare and Medicaid (42 C.F.R. §482.13).

Since few correctional facilities are participants in the Medicare or Medicaid systems, the rules established by CMS concerning the use of restraint and seclusion had little impact on the use of seclusion or restraint for mental health care purposes in correctional systems. As a result, many correctional health care systems have not developed policies, procedures, or practices that are consistent with the current community practice. In addition, the frequent lack of meaningful external review or oversight in many correctional facilities regarding their mental health care practices has contributed to correctional facilities not keeping pace with prevailing community standards. When correctional health care systems use seclusion or restraint for health care purposes, they should be held to a similar standard of care as community health facilities, just as correctional facilities are not permitted to perform intrusive medical interventions unless they are done in a manner consistent with the community standard in appropriate health care settings.

General Principles

General issues, indications and contraindications for the mental health use of seclusion or restraint in non-correctional mental health facilities, and specific techniques are summarized in Appendix I. When seclusion or restraint is used as a mental health intervention, the principles described in Appendix I almost always apply, with a few exceptions that will be addressed below. The exceptions are related to certain differences between correctional and community healthcare settings.

Issues Unique to the Correctional Setting

Location

The first major issue specific to the correctional setting involves the location where the incarcerated person (hereinafter referred to as an "inmate") is secluded or restrained for mental health purposes. This setting in jails and prisons nationwide may appropriately include hospitals, infirmaries and/or special housing units (often referred to as residential treatment units, intermediate care units, special needs units, extended outpatient units, etc.) within the correctional setting for inmates with serious mental illnesses.

When an inmate is secluded or restrained in a hospital setting, the rules promulgated by CMS should be followed, regardless of where the hospital is located or what agency administratively operates the hospital.

When an inmate is secluded or restrained in a non-hospital setting, the seclusion or restraint should nonetheless occur within a health care setting. The most common such setting is the prison or jail infirmary, which is generally characterized by 24 hour nursing coverage, whose mission is to provide health care assessments/treatment for inmates requiring a more structured medical setting than is available elsewhere in the correctional institution. The guidelines relevant to the design of the seclusion or restraint room in hospitals are applicable (see Appendix I), although the security requirements of a correctional facility will also impact the physical characteristics of the seclusion or restraint room.

The use of seclusion for clinical reasons is unusual in a correctional infirmary setting because it is common practice, due to security regulations, for an inmate to be essentially locked down (i.e., secluded for custody purposes) in his/her infirmary cell throughout the course of treatment, which is generally short-term in nature (i.e., less than two weeks). However, some states license correctional infirmaries and specifically prohibit such a routine practice, although exceptions are allowed. Under such circumstances, the guidelines described in this resource document relevant to seclusion would be applicable or the correctional facility would at least need to be compliant with the relevant licensure requirements.

Seclusion or restraint in special housing units for inmates with mental illness can be implemented in a clinically appropriate way, although it is often more logistically difficulty to do so because of the physical plant of many of these housing units. In addition, many special housing units for inmates with mental illness are not staffed around the clock by nursing staff. The guidelines relevant to the use of seclusion or restraint in correctional infirmaries are applicable to these special housing units. In other words, if seclusion or restraint is used in these special housing units, staffing requirements such as 24-hour nursing will need to be available in order to implement the relevant policies and procedures.

It is not clinically appropriate to use locked down units (housing unit where inmates are generally locked in their cell for 22–23 hours per day such for disciplinary or administrative reasons) such as administrative, disciplinary, or punitive segregation housing units for inmates with mental illnesses who require the use of seclusion or restraint for clinical reasons. These units do not provide a supportive or therapeutic environment and the environmental conditions often exacerbate the clinical condition of the inmate requiring seclusion or restraint. In addition, these units are not adequately staffed by nursing or other health care staff for monitoring and treatment purposes.

Property

Unless clinically contraindicated, which should be infrequent, inmates secluded or restrained should have a mattress, blanket and clothing. The nonflammable mattress should be constructed of durable foam and not fiber or other substance, which the patient could conceivably use for self-harm purposes. Clothing may consist of paper gowns or so-called "suicide smocks," which are essentially tear resistant blankets that are designed to be worn as clothing.

Timeframes

As described in Appendix I, the Centers for Medicare and Medicaid Services (CMS), has defined rules for the use of seclusion and restraint in facilities that participate in Medicare and Medicaid (42 C.F.R. §482.13) that has provided a framework for a national standard for the use of seclusion and restraint in psychiatric facilities. CMS guidelines specify that, absent immediate need to protect the patient or others from substantial harm, a physician or "licensed independent practitioner" (LIP) must be the one to order and monitor restraint and seclusion.

The major departure from the guidelines summarized in Appendix I involves the time parameters related to the initial face-to-face assessment by an appropriately credentialed mental health clinician. This resource document recommends that the initial face-to-face assessment by a licensed independent professional occur within four hours of the actual seclusion or restraint. All physicians and other licensed independent professionals (LIPs) should be appropriately trained in the use of seclusion and restraint. If the LIP is not a physician, consultation should be obtained by the LIP with a physician, appropriately trained in the use of seclusion or restraints, within the same four-hour timeframe.

Face-to-face assessments should occur at least every 12 hours after the initial assessment, and should be performed by an appropriately trained and credentialed physician, LIP, or registered nurse. If the assessment is not performed by a qualified physician, one should be consulted. A qualified physician should do a face-to-face assessment at least every 24 hours if the inmate remains in restraints or seclusion. Very brief periods of release do not reset the "clock" for assessments. Consultation by another psychiatrist, when feasible, should be obtained for inmates requiring prolonged periods (e.g., >24 hours) of seclusion or restraint.

A variety of restraint devices exist on the market. Steel restraints (e.g., handcuffs), although acceptable for use when the indications are custody issues, should rarely be used for mental health purposes. The use of a device commonly referred to as a "restraint chair" is much more frequent in correctional setting as compared to community hospital settings. The main advantage of this device (i.e., mobility, which allows the restraint to occur in many different settings in contrast to just being limited to an appropriately constructed seclusion or restraint room) is also its major disadvantage. Specifically, the restraint chair is often used in a housing unit where the environment is not supportive and staff are not trained or experienced with the use of restraint. This is one of the reasons that the use of restraints for mental health purposes in a correctional setting should occur within a health-care setting in contrast to a non-healthcare custody setting such as an administrative segregation housing unit. Proper procedures are less likely to be followed in such circumstances, which increases the likelihood of an adverse outcome.

Policies and procedures concerning the use of seclusion or restraint for inmates with mental illness need to be in written form as part of the health care policy and procedures manual. The initial order for the use of seclusion or restraint should be obtained within one hour of the use of seclusion or restraint from a licensed independent practitioner, preferably a physician, although seclusion or restraint can be initiated by nursing staff under emergency conditions prior to receiving the actual order from a LIP. Training and re-training of health care and correctional staffs that will be involved in the seclusion or restraint procedure is required. This is particularly crucial in terms of the technique of actually restraining an inmate and the subsequent observations/interventions that are required, such as range of motion exercises and clinical assessments.

Logbooks should also be maintained of the use of seclusion or restraint for mental health purposes, which will facilitate quality improvement reviews. The logbooks should identify the inmate being secluded or restrained, reason for such intervention, duration of the intervention, and other pertinent data.

References

American Psychiatric Association: Psychiatric Services in Jails and Prisons, 2nd Edition. Washington, DC, American Psychiatric Association, 2000

American Psychiatric Association, American Psychiatric Nurses Association, National Association of Psychiatric Health Systems: Learning From Each Other: Success Stories and Ideas for Reducing Restraint/Seclusion in Behavioral Health. Arlington, VA, American Psychiatric Association, 2003

Huckshorn KA: Six Core Strategies for Reducing Seclusion and Restraint Use. Draft Example: Policy and Procedure on Debriefing for Seclusion and Restraint Reduction Project. Alexandria, VA, National Technical Assistance Center for State Mental Health Planning, 2006. Available at: http://www.nasmhpd.org/general_files/publications/ntac_pubs/Debriefing%20p%20and%20p%20with%20cover%207-05.pdf.

National Association of State Mental Health Program Directors Medical Directors Council: Reducing the Use of Seclusion and Restraint Part II: Findings, Principles, and Recommendations for Special Needs Populations. Alexandria, VA, National Association of State Mental Health Program Directors Medical Directors Council, March 2001. Available at: http://www.nasmhpd.org/docs/publications/archiveDocs/2001/Seclusion_Restraint_2.pdf. Accessed June 20, 2006.

National Commission on Correctional Health Care: Standards for Health Services in Jails. Chicago, IL, National Commission on Correctional Health Care, 2003a
National Commission on Correctional Health Care: Standards for Health Services in Prisons. Chicago, IL, National Commission on Correctional Health Care, 2003b
National Technical Assistance Center for State Mental Health Planning: Violence and Coercion and Mental Health Settings: Eliminating the Use of Seclusion and Restraint. Networks (Special Edition). Alexandria, VA, National Association of State Mental Health Program Directors, Summer/Fall 2002. Available at: http://www.nasmhpd.org/general_files/publications/ntac_pubs/networks/SummerFall2002.pdf. Accessed June 20, 2006.

Appendix I

In 1999, the Health Care Financing Administration (HCFA), now called the Centers for Medicare and Medicaid Services (CMS), defined rules for the use of seclusion and restraint in facilities that participate in Medicare and Medicaid (42 C.F.R. §482.13). The final rule states that restraint use must be in accordance with safe and appropriate restraining techniques; and selected only when other less restrictive measures have been found to be ineffective to protect the patient or others from harm.

Other indications for seclusion and restraint include the following:

1. To prevent serious disruption of the treatment program/milieu or significant damage to the physical environment, and
2. For treatment as part of an appropriately approved, initiated, and monitored plan of behavior therapy.

CMS interpretive guidelines make it clear that for restraint used for behavioral/psychiatric purposes "it is important to note that these requirements are not specific to any treatment setting, but to the situation the restraint is being used to address. Further, the decision to use a restraint is driven not by diagnosis, but by comprehensive individual assessment that concludes that for this patient at this time, the use of less intrusive measures poses a greater risk than the risk of using a restraint or seclusion" (Department of Health and Human Services [DHHS] Health Care Financing Administration [HCFA], June 2000. Medicare State Operations Manual, Provider Certification. Appendix A: Interpretive Guidelines and Survey Procedures–Hospitals).

Some reasons to consider seclusion or restraint include, but are not limited to the following:

• Signs or symptoms associated with significant danger to others, including threats and intimidation of staff or other patients, which are not immediately manageable by less restrictive means;

- Severe agitation for which medication is inadequate, unavailable (e.g., because of patient allergy or adverse effects), or has not yet taken effect;
- Disruption of the clinical or residential milieu sufficient to interfere with the rights or well-being of patients or staff, for which less restrictive interventions are either inadequate or truly not feasible (that is, beyond mere staff or patient inconvenience);
- Dangerous, agitated, or disruptive behavior whose origins are unclear, and for which seclusion or restraint is likely to be safer than medication or other measures because of insufficient knowledge about the patient's medical condition;
- Intractable behavior or impulse control problems for which a specific form of seclusion or restraint is part of an approved behavior modification program;
- Repeated, or repeatedly threatened, significant damage to others' property for which less restrictive measures are inadequate or not feasible; and
- Situations in which immediate control of the patient is necessary to protect the patient's or others' significant interests, but for which less restrictive measures are inadequate or not feasible (e.g., controlling severe agitation or manic behavior while waiting for calming medication to take effect).

Some reasons to consider not ordering seclusion or restraint include, but are not limited to, the following:

- A patient's marked panic at being restrained;
- A patient's marked proneness to claustrophobia in a seclusion room;
- Unavailability of sufficient qualified staff to monitor the secluded or restrained patient (including constant monitoring of a suicidal patient in seclusion or a patient whose general medical condition is unclear);
- Unavailability of a seclusion room which is sufficiently free of ways in which the patient may injure himself;
- In contemplating use for behavioral programs, insufficient consideration by appropriately trained and experienced professionals of the risks and benefits of seclusion or restraint, and consideration of other available measures; and
- Staff requests for seclusion or restraint that the ordering clinician believes may be related to neglect, abuse, insufficient consideration of alternative measures, or mere staff convenience.

Seclusion or restraint for intimidation of others or milieu disruption requires more discrimination than that for actual assault or agitation. Behaviors such as screaming, public masturbation, intrusiveness, or fecal smearing may constitute indications for restrictive measures, but the extent to which they actually affect others or interfere with their care requires careful consideration. Seclusion or restraint for protective reasons (as contrasted with approved behavioral programs) is not primary treatment in itself, and does not take the place of efforts to understand and address the causes of the aberrant behavior.

In most uses of seclusion or restraint, the staff should have considered or tried less restrictive means of control, such as verbal, environmental, or pharmacological interventions. Staff should be trained, encouraged, and supervised to understand and engage with their patients. The treatment environment and individual treatment programs should "fit," and be able to tolerate, the symptoms and behaviors expected of patients with various disorders common to that unit.

The use of medication as an alternative to seclusion or restraint is different from its use in treating underlying symptoms or disorders. The latter should not be seen as, nor compared to, a form of "restraint." Drugs are considered a restraint under CMS regulations only if the drug used is not a standard treatment for the patient's medical or psychiatric disorder. Standard treatments include use of the medication for its labeled indications, use of the medication follows national practice standards, and use of the medication is ordered by the prescriber for the patient's individualized needs. A medication that is not being used as a standard treatment for the patient's medical or psychiatric condition, and that results in controlling the patient's behavior and/or in restricting his or her freedom of movement would be a drug used as a restraint under the regulations. (Interpretive Guidelines §482.13[f][1], http://cms.hhs.gov/manuals/Downloads/som107ap_a_hospitals.pdf [accessed 09/16/2006].) Context and individual patient circumstances should be carefully considered in the weighing of risk and benefit when using a drug to treat the symptoms underlying episodes of patient aggression.

The use of seclusion and restraint as part of an approved and monitored behavior treatment program should be used infrequently. Such use differs from the other indications in that it is planned beforehand and monitored so as to attempt long-term change in the patient's behavior or psychopathology rather than simply addressing immediate concerns.

Contraindications

Seclusion or restraint may be contraindicated in patients with certain clinical condition (such as unstable medical status, known or suspected intolerance for immobility, conditions in which restraint positioning is contraindicated, some dementias and deliria, some paranoid conditions and anxiety syndromes). In addition, some posttraumatic syndromes (including those following torture, kidnapping or severe sexual abuse) can increase a patient's vulnerability to traumatic re-experiencing or sensory deprivation, making either seclusion or restraint (or both) very difficult to tolerate.

Seclusion as a purely punitive response is contraindicated in clinical settings. Similarly, patients should not be secluded solely for the comfort or convenience of the staff, for mere mild obnoxiousness, rudeness or other unpleasantness by the patient to others that does not significantly interfere with their rights or treatment.

Seclusion Room Design

Clinicians and direct care staff should be aware of the real and potential hazards of seclusion rooms. Poorly designed ones can be relatively dangerous to patients, particularly those left unattended. Suicide and other harm is more likely in seclusion rooms than in many other locations on inpatient units, for reasons related partially to architecture and partially to the characteristics and higher acuity of patients confined there. Useful guidelines have been published by the National Association of Psychiatric Health Systems which address such things as fixtures, temperature control, lighting, and patient visibility in seclusion rooms and restraint settings (Guidelines for Built Environment of Behavioral Health Facilities, last accessed May 27, 2006 via www.naphs.org).

In general, the room should be empty, with a high ceiling (>9 feet) and fixtures that are recessed sufficiently that they cannot be either damaged or used by the patient for self-harm. Temperature and lighting (with security fixtures) should be adequate, with sufficient privacy but good access to the nursing station. The room should be without sharp corners. Walls and ceilings should be made of material that cannot be gouged out or picked apart by patients who are intent on harming themselves. Sheet rock, plaster board, and ordinary tufted mats, for example, are not acceptable. Padded walls can be used, provided the integrity of the material used is high and the surfaces clean; there are insufficient data to warrant specific materials recommendations, except to say that they must take into account foreseeable risks to the patients who will be confined.

The door should open outward, so that the patient cannot barricade himself inside. Protuberances, such as knobs, fixtures, or ledges, should not be present in the room. Each room must permit staff observation of the patient while still providing for patient privacy. Windows, which are recommended for lighting and to reduce isolation, must be constructed of Plexiglas®- or Lexan®-like material (or otherwise adequately shielded) and take safety and privacy into account. The mattress should be the only furnishing in the room; a bed, even when bolted to the floor, poses a number of dangers. The mattress should be constructed of durable foam, not fibers or other substances which the patient might use to hang or otherwise injure himself, and should not be flammable nor emit noxious fumes when heated. Any lock on a seclusion room must be controlled by staff at the door location and must unlock when released by the staff person.

Restraint room design is very similar to the seclusion room, with the exception of a bolted bed specifically designed for restraint purposes.

Timeframes

Initiation of a restraint procedure or placement of a patient in seclusion is usually an emergency procedure carried out by nursing and other professional staff in accordance with established hospital policy. CMS guidelines specify that, absent immediate need to protect the patient or others from substantial harm, a physician or "licensed independent practitioner" (LIP) must be the one to order and monitor restraint and seclusion. CMS describes such clinicians as being trained in emergency care techniques and licensed by their state to write such orders. According to CMS, a patient should be seen face-to-face by the physician or licensed independent practitioner within one hour after initiation of restraint or seclusion. If a patient is released from seclusion before the initial assessment, the LIP must still render an evaluation within that first hour's time. The behavioral standard also requires that written orders for physical restraint or seclusion be limited to four hours for adults, two hours for children and adolescents aged 9 to 17, and one hour for patients less than nine years old. After the first specified time period, new orders for further restraint or seclusion (of similar duration) are required, which may be given on the basis of information conveyed by telephone, without face- to-face evaluations, and repeated for up to 24 hours. (DHHS, HCFA [42 C.F.R. 482]. Medicare and Medicaid Programs: Conditions of Participation: Patient's Rights: Interim Final Rule. Federal Register 64:36069–36089. 1999. See State Operations Manual Appendix A–Survey Protocol, Regulations and Interpretive Guidelines for Hospitals [Rev. 1, 05–21–04] Sections 482.13[e] and 482.13[f] http://cms.hhs.gov/manuals/Downloads/som107ap_a_hospitals.pdf [accessed 09/16/2006].)

Some patients require face-to-face visits more frequently than others. Examples include those with significant concurrent medical problems, dementia or delirium, and significant intoxications, and restraint situations in which hyperthermia may occur. Some patients must be restrained or secluded for more than 24 hours. In such instances, a senior medical administrator, such as the chief physician of the institution or a qualified designee should review the treatment plan and concur that additional restraint or seclusion is necessary. In general medical facilities with psychiatric divisions, this person may be the chief psychiatrist.

It is recommended that orders be time and behavior specific, with a stated goal (e.g., "four-point restraints until patient is no longer agitated and combative, up to one hour"). Standing orders for restraint or seclusion should not be allowed. The clinician must document in the patient's record the failure of less restrictive alternatives, or why they are inappropriate to attempt, and the justification for continued seclusion or restraint. This decision should take into account the mental and physical status of the patient, his or her degree of agitation, the potential adverse effects of seclusion (both physical and emotional), and relevant other factors. Debriefing at the end of the episode, of staff at least and the patient when feasible, is important and should be well documented.

Restraint and Seclusion Techniques

Although there are no specific national protocols for restraint and seclusion technique, there are a number of common threads among acceptable procedures. First, the techniques practiced within a particular facility should be rehearsed and approved by the staff, including the relevant chief of service. If a particular technique and modality, such as four-point leather restraints, is viewed as usual practice, that should be specifically noted in the facility policy manual. Details of the technique should be disseminated to members of the clinical and direct care staff as part of service training. Written instructions, photographs, and videotapes are desirable.

Even patients at low risk of suicide should always be searched before being placed in seclusion. Agitated or violent patients may become self-destructive or self-mutilating when isolated.

Any need for seclusion or restraint should be part of the patient's treatment plan. With regard to the treatment plan, however, one should recognize that seclusion or restraint are usually emergency procedures which cannot be anticipated in many treatment plans unless there is a history of previous restrictive needs. That having been said, when clinically feasible, patients should be informed about restrictive procedures and policies during the admission and orientation process.

Once the decision has been made to proceed with seclusion or restraint, a seclusion or restraint "leader" is chosen from available staff. When feasible or necessary for safety, the team should consist of at least one trained staff member per limb, including the head. Staff should convey an air of united confidence, calm, and measured control, reflecting a professional approach to a routine and familiar procedure. A seclusion monitor should be designated to clear other patients and physical obstructions. The monitor should remain clear of the physical activity to objectively observe the process and note any injuries or difficulties. This promotes accurate critique after the event.

Confrontation of the patient should begin with a clear communication of purpose and rationale for the seclusion or restraint. The patient is given a few clear behavioral options without undue verbal threat or provocation. For example, the patient may be told that his or her behavior is out of control and that a period of seclusion is required to help him regain control, then the patient is told to walk quietly to the seclusion room accompanied by staff.

This is not the time for negotiation or psychodynamic interpretation. Since the decision for seclusion or restraint has already been made, any further negotiation is superfluous, and may to lead to more disruptive behavior and/or aggravation of violence.

At this point the team should position itself around the patient in such a manner as to allow rapid access to the patient's extremities if necessary. If the patient does not do as he/she is told, then at a predetermined signal from the leader, physical force commences, using techniques previously learned and practiced for their effectiveness and low likelihood of injury to either patient or staff. Each staff member seizes and controls the appropriate part of the patient and each limb is restrained at the joint. The patient's head should be controlled to prevent biting. With the patient completely controlled on the ground, additional staff may be called to secure the limbs and prepare to move the patient to the seclusion room or apply mechanical restraints. In very violent cases, staff may have to carry the patient into the seclusion room. This involves lifting the patient in the recumbent position with his/her arms pinned to the sides, legs held tightly at the knees, head controlled, and force applied uniformly to support the back, hips and legs.

If the patient is taken to seclusion, he/she should be positioned on his back with the head toward the door. An assessment should be made regarding whether or not to remove his or her clothing and put on a seclusion-safe hospital gown. Special attention should be paid to rings, belts, shoelaces and other potentially injurious objects. Medication may be given while the patient is physically restrained. The staff then exits in a coordinated fashion, one at a time, releasing the legs before the arms.

In acute restraint, a face down posture is often safer because the patient is less apt to bite or aspirate, although the risk of positional asphyxia is increased. Monitoring breathing adequacy is critical to any restraint process. This is a particular risk in obese patients or those with a medical condition that can obstruct breathing (such as a large goiter). Such patients should be restrained face up. Staff should also be cautious about placing knees on any patient's back, which can compromise breathing.

A debriefing follows each seclusion or restraint maneuver to review the technique and progress of the event and allow release of staff members' feelings and tension. The event should also be discussed openly among the patient population to uncover and allay their concerns associated with both the patient's behavior and the staff's use of force. The patient should also be asked later about the experience, including whether it contributed to or worsened his or her sense of control. The entire seclusion or restraint episode should be scrupulously documented, in detail, in the patient's chart and on appropriate facility forms.

Observation and Patient Protection

Patients in restraint that prevents their moving about (such as "4-point" restraints), is combined with seclusion, may compromise breathing or circulation, or makes them vulnerable to abuse by other patients should be continuously observed. Continuous monitoring is also recommended for patients in seclusion, especially those who are intoxicated, psychotic, severely depressed, reasonably likely to be suicidal, known to be prone to self-injury, or unfamiliar to staff. In no event should a secluded patient be monitored less than every 15 minutes.

Documentation of observations should be continuous and contemporaneous (i.e., done at the time of the observation). Staff should be cautioned not to fill in monitoring checklists in advance, nor to complete them all at once at the end of a shift or monitoring period.

Continuous video monitoring of patients in seclusion is common, but should not be the only form of monitoring unless a staff person is specifically assigned to watch the screen continuously and the screen itself should be placed in an area conducive to patient privacy. Simply having the screen in a nursing area and expecting staff to check it is not sufficient.

Documentation of visual observation (not the same as periodic assessments, below) should note the time and identity of the observer, and comment briefly on the patient's general appearance, behavior, and whether or not any problems or injuries are apparent (such as gross indications of exhaustion, overheating, or soiling).

Care of Patients in Seclusion or Restraints

When agitated patients are approached in the seclusion room, the same number of staff should enter the room as were required to safely control the patient earlier (e.g., one for each extremity). Once the patient is calm, and after considering staff safety, direct observation may be made with the seclusion room door open. This allows for better observation and communication, and decreases the restrictiveness of the intervention.

To ensure the continuation of adequate circulation, nursing staff should physically check each extremity every fifteen (15) minutes for at least the first two hours of restraint. Every two hours, nursing staff should perform an assessment of the patient, including condition of skin and circulation, need for toileting, personal hygiene procedures, and proper application of the restraint. Documentation of the two-hour evaluations should summarize the patient's overall physical condition, general behavior, and response to counseling/interviews. Vital signs should be taken at least every eight hours.

Range of motion exercises should be performed every two hours unless the patient is too agitated or assaultive to safely remove the restraints. For range of motion exercises, restraints on each extremity shall be removed, one at a time. Performance of range of motion exercises shall be clearly documented and as well as the patient's behavior, respiration, and responsiveness. If range-of-motion exercises are not performed, nursing staff shall clearly document the reason.

Fluids and nourishment should also be provided every two hours except during hours of sleep. The patient's head and shoulders should be elevated, if needed, while being fed or receiving fluids to reduce the risk of aspiration.

Toileting of the patient should be provided at least every four hours, and more often if necessary. If the toilet facilities are outside the restraint or seclusion area, and/or safety concerns suggest that release would be unnecessarily dangerous, a urinal or bed pan should be used with appropriate considerations of both privacy and safety.

Fluids are vital for patients in restraint or seclusion, particularly those who perspire profusely or are otherwise prone to dehydration. Documentation of fluid intake, though often difficult with regressed patients, is required.

Meals should be brought to the patient at regular intervals when the other patients are served. All utensils should be blunt and unbreakable; plastic knives and forks can be used as weapons. Remember that some foods can be used as a weapon. In certain rare instances, such as with severely regressed patients, a food tray may be placed within the patient's reach without a staff person being present. (The rationale for this solitary meal procedure should be documented in detail in nursing notes; meals should be a time of interaction between patient and staff whenever reasonably possible.)

Patients in restraint and seclusion may exhaust themselves from the physical activity of pushing or pulling against restraint devices or walking or running around the seclusion room. Attention must be given to the possibility of dangerous fatigue or dehydration, especially in older, obese, or medically compromised patients, those whose medications make them prone to poor temperature regulation, and those in high-temperature environments.

Some patients soil themselves in the process of menstruation, incontinence, or vomiting, or have other conditions that create some level of embarrassment or repugnance to themselves or others. While rarely a dangerous condition, such conditions often cause feelings of humiliation and avoidance by others. It is important that such patients not be ignored or neglected, and that the problem is handled without unnecessary stigmatization.

Both seclusion and restraint can contribute to worsening of psychiatric symptoms, especially anxiety, isolation, and psychosis. Some level of sensory stimulation is inherent in most restrictive measures. This should be considered when discussing the possibility of future restriction upon admission and when choosing a mode of restriction when the patient's behavior requires it. The emotional impact of seclusion, for example, may be discussed with the patient, when feasible, during the experience and may be one of the topics addressed in patient debriefing after release. Such discussions may help reduce adverse effects and prevent painful memories.

It is very important not to underestimate patients' abilities to find ways to harm themselves while in seclusion. The danger can be mitigated with careful attention to the construction of the room, attention to patients' clothing and possessions while confined, and by close staff monitoring.

Decisions and Procedures for Removal From Seclusion and Restraint

Patients should be released from seclusion or restraint when the goals of the intervention have been achieved and safety for the patient and others can be reasonably assured. In some cases, the patient's ability to control his/her behavior can be inferred from observations during seclusion or restraint. In others, risk must be estimated in other ways. Each time staff enter or otherwise interact with the patient (e.g., for feeding, bathing or examining), the patient's behavior, responses to requests or demands, and verbal interchange may offer important clues to his affect and impulse control.

Removal from restraint and/or seclusion does not have to be abrupt. Graduated steps are often safer, and allow staff to judge the safety and appropriateness of further decreasing the restriction. Restraints may be partially removed at first, or the seclusion room door opened while the patient is closely monitored.

Staff Training

Staff should be trained in the necessary safety precautions for all secluded or restrained patients, not just those with known or suspected contraindications. A training and certification process should be in place, with documentation that every staff member who will ever participate in a restraint or seclusion episode is recertified annually. The training should include hands-on experience with experienced instructors.

APPENDIX 7

APA Official Actions

Position Statement on Capital Punishment:
*Adoption of AMA Statements
on Capital Punishment*

Approved by the Board of Trustees, July 2008

Approved by the Assembly, May 2008

"Policy documents are approved by the APA Assembly
and Board of Trustees.... These are...position statements
that define APA official policy on specific subjects..."

– APA Operations Manual

AMA Policy E-2.06 Capital Punishment

An individual's opinion on capital punishment is the personal moral decision of the individual. A physician, as a member of a profession dedicated to preserving life when there is hope of doing so, should not be a participant in a legally authorized execution. Physician participation in execution is defined generally as actions which would fall into one or more of the fol-

---

Issued July 1980. Updated June 1994 based on the report "Physician Participation in Capital Punishment," adopted December 1992, (JAMA. 1993; 270:365–368); updated June 1996 based on the report "Physician Participation in Capital Punishment: Evaluations of Prisoner Competence to be Executed; Treatment to Restore Competence to be Executed," adopted in June 1995; Updated December 1999; and Updated June 2000 based on the report "Defining Physician Participation in State Executions," adopted June 1998.

lowing categories: (1) an action which would directly cause the death of the condemned; (2) an action which would assist, supervise, or contribute to the ability of another individual to directly cause the death of the condemned; (3) an action which could automatically cause an execution to be carried out on a condemned prisoner.

Physician participation in an execution includes, but is not limited to, the following actions: prescribing or administering tranquilizers and other psychotropic agents and medications that are part of the execution procedure; monitoring vital signs on site or remotely (including monitoring electrocardiograms); attending or observing an execution as a physician; and rendering of technical advice regarding execution. In the case where the method of execution is lethal injection, the following actions by the physician would also constitute physician participation in execution: selecting injection sites; starting intravenous lines as a port for a lethal injection device; prescribing, preparing, administering, or supervising injection drugs or their doses or types; inspecting, testing, or maintaining lethal injection devices; and consulting with or supervising lethal injection personnel.

The following actions do not constitute physician participation in execution: (1) testifying as to medical history and diagnoses or mental state as they relate to competence to stand trial, testifying as to relevant medical evidence during trial, testifying as to medical aspects of aggravating or mitigating circumstances during the penalty phase of a capital case, or testifying as to medical diagnoses as they relate to the legal assessment of competence for execution; (2) certifying death, provided that the condemned has been declared dead by another person; (3) witnessing an execution in a totally nonprofessional capacity; (4) witnessing an execution at the specific voluntary request of the condemned person, provided that the physician observes the execution in a nonprofessional capacity; and (5) relieving the acute suffering of a condemned person while awaiting execution, including providing tranquilizers at the specific voluntary request of the condemned person to help relieve pain or anxiety in anticipation of the execution.

Physicians should not determine legal competence to be executed. A physician's medical opinion should be merely one aspect of the information taken into account by a legal decision maker such as a judge or hearing officer. When a condemned prisoner has been declared incompetent to be executed, physicians should not treat the prisoner for the purpose of restoring competence unless a commutation order is issued before treatment begins. The task of re-evaluating the prisoner should be performed by an independent physician examiner. If the incompetent prisoner is undergoing extreme suffering as a result of psychosis or any other illness, medical intervention intended to mitigate the level of suffering is ethically permissible. No physician should be compelled to participate in the process of establishing a prisoner's competence or be involved with treatment of an incompetent, condemned prisoner if such activity is contrary to the physician's personal beliefs. Under those circumstances, physicians should be permitted to transfer care of the prisoner to another physician.

Organ donation by condemned prisoners is permissible only if (1) the decision to donate was made before the prisoner's conviction, (2) the donated tissue is harvested after the prisoner has been pronounced dead and the body removed from the death chamber, and (3) physicians do not provide advice on modifying the method of execution for any individual to facilitate donation.

APPENDIX 8

APA Official Actions

Position Statement on Atypical Antipsychotic Medications

Approved by the Board of Trustees, September 2009

Approved by the Assembly, May 2009

> "Policy documents are approved by the APA Assembly and Board of Trustees....These are...position statements that define APA official policy on specific subjects..."
>
> *– APA Operations Manual*

Given the current state of knowledge, it is our opinion that the new generation of antipsychotic medications (except clozapine) need to be made available as first-line treatments for appropriate individuals throughout all systems of care. Similarly, clozapine needs to be made available for individuals with treatment refractory psychotic disorders. Access to these medications needs to be made available in all systems of health care and by all public and private insurers including all jails, prisons and youth services facilities.

APA Official Actions

Position Statement on Access to Care for Transgender and Gender Variant Individuals

Approved by the Board of Trustees, July 2012

Approved by the Assembly, May 2012

> "Policy documents are approved by the APA Assembly and Board of Trustees....These are...position statements that define APA official policy on specific subjects..."
>
> – *APA Operations Manual*

Issue: Significant and long-standing medical and psychiatric literature exists that demonstrates clear benefits of medical and surgical interventions to assist gender variant individuals seeking transition. However, private and public insurers often do not offer, or may specifically exclude, coverage for medically necessary treatments for gender transition. Access to medical care (both medical and surgical) positively impacts the mental health of transgender and gender variant individuals.

The APA's vision statement includes the phrase: "Its vision is a society that has available, accessible quality psychiatric diagnosis and treatment," yet currently, transgender and gender variant individuals frequently lack available and accessible treatment. In addition, APA's values include the following points:

Authors: Jack Drescher, M.D., Ellen Haller, M.D., APA Caucus of Lesbian, Gay and Bisexual Psychiatrists.

- best standards of clinical practice
- patient-focused treatment decisions
- scientifically established principles of treatment
- advocacy for patients

Transgender and gender variant individuals currently lack access to the best standards of clinical practice, frequently do not have the opportunity to pursue patient-focused treatment decisions, do not receive scientifically established treatment and could benefit significantly from APA's advocacy.

APA Position

Therefore, the American Psychiatric Association:

1. **Recognizes that appropriately evaluated transgender and gender variant individuals can benefit greatly from medical and surgical gender transition treatments.**
2. **Advocates for removal of barriers to care and supports both public and private health insurance coverage for gender transition treatment.**
3. **Opposes categorical exclusions of coverage for such medically necessary treatment when prescribed by a physician.**

Background to the Position Statement

Transgender and gender variant people are frequently denied medical, surgical and psychiatric care related to gender transition despite significant evidence that appropriately evaluated individuals benefit from such care. It is often asserted that the DSM (and ICD) diagnoses provide the only pathways to insurance reimbursement for transgender individuals seeking medical assistance. However, to date, the APA has issued no treatment guidelines for gender identity disorder (GID) in either children or adults. This omission is in contrast to an increasing proliferation of APA practice guidelines for other DSM diagnoses (Drescher 2010).

The absence of a formal APA opinion about treatment of a diagnosis of its own creation has contributed to an ongoing problem of many health care insurers and other third party payers claiming that hormonal treatment and sex reassignment surgery (SRS) are "experimental treatments," "elective treatments," or "not medically necessary," and, therefore, not reimbursable or covered under most insurance plans. The lack of consistency in how a transgender condition is defined by some institutions further marginalizes these individuals based on their subjective, surgical and hormonal status (Rosenblum 2000). In addition, treatment is not always accessible to wards of governmental agencies, such as transgender and gender variant individuals in foster care and prison systems. In other words, the presence of the GID diagnosis in the DSM has not served its intended purpose of creating greater access to care—one of the major arguments for diagnostic retention (Drescher 2010).

Lack of access to care adversely impacts the mental health of transgender and gender variant people, and both hormonal and surgical treatment have been shown to be efficacious in these individuals (De Cuypere et al. 2005; Institute of Medicine 2011; Newfield et al. 2006; Smith et al. 2005; World Professional Association for Transgender Health 2011). Practice guidelines have been developed based on peer-reviewed scientific studies and are published and available for clinicians to access (Hembree et al. 2009; UCSF Center of Excellence for Transgender Health 2011; World Professional Association for Transgender Health 2011). The American Medical Association and the American Psychological Association both have position statements stating the critical importance of access to care for transgender and gender variant individuals (American Medical Association 2011; American Psychological Association 2008).

References

American Medical Association: Removing Financial Barriers to Care for Transgender Patients. Available at: http://www.ama-assn.org/ama/pub/about-ama/our-people/member-groups-sections/glbt-advisory-committee/ama-policy-regarding-sexual-orientation.page? Accessed May 16, 2011.

American Psychological Association: APA Policy Statement: Transgender, Gender Identity, and Gender Expression Non-Discrimination. Washington, DC, American Psychological Association, 2008. Available at: http://www.apa.org/about/policy/transgender.aspx. Accessed May 16, 2011.

De Cuypere G, T'Sjoen G, Beerten R, et al: Sexual and physical health after sex reassignment surgery. Arch Sex Behav 34(6):679–690, 2005 16362252

Drescher J: Queer diagnoses: parallels and contrasts in the history of homosexuality, gender variance, and the Diagnostic and Statistical Manual (DSM). Arch Sex Behav 39(2):427–460, 2010 19838785

Hembree WC, Cohen-Kettenis P, Delemarre-van de Waal HA, et al: Endocrine treatment of transsexual persons: an Endocrine Society clinical practice guideline. J Clin Endocrinol Metab 94(9):3132–3154, 2009 19509099

Institute of Medicine: The Health of Lesbian, Gay, Bisexual, and Transgender People: Building a Foundation for Better Understanding. Washington, DC, The National Academies Press, 2011. Available at: http://www.iom.edu/Reports/2011/The-Health-of-Lesbian-Gay-Bisexual-and-Transgender-People.aspx. Accessed May 16, 2011.

Newfield E, Hart S, Dibble S, et al: Female-to-male transgender quality of life. Qual Life Res 15(9):1447–1457, 2006 16758113

Rosenblum D: "Trapped" in Sing Sing: transgendered prisoners caught in the gender binarism. Paper 207. New York, Pace Law Faculty Publications, 2000

Smith YL, Van Goozen SH, Kuiper AJ, et al: Sex reassignment: outcomes and predictors of treatment for adolescent and adult transsexuals. Psychol Med 35(1):89–99, 2005 15842032

UCSF Center of Excellence for Transgender Health: Primary Care Protocol for Transgender Patient Care, April 2011. Available at: http://transhealth.ucsf.edu/trans?page=protocol-00-00. Accessed May 16, 2011.

World Professional Association for Transgender Health: Standards of Care. Available at: http://www.wpath.org/publications_standards.cfm. Accessed May 16, 2011.

APPENDIX 10

APA Official Actions

Position Statement on Segregation of Prisoners With Mental Illness

Approved by the Board of Trustees, December 2012

Approved by the Assembly, November 2012

> "Policy documents are approved by the APA Assembly and Board of Trustees....These are...position statements that define APA official policy on specific subjects..."
>
> – *APA Operations Manual*

Prolonged segregation of adult inmates with serious mental illness, with rare exceptions, should be avoided due to the potential for harm to such inmates. If an inmate with serious mental illness is placed in segregation, out-of-cell structured therapeutic activities (i.e., mental health/psychiatric treatment) in appropriate programming space and adequate unstructured out-of-cell time should be permitted. Correctional mental health authorities should work closely with administrative custody staff to maximize access to clinically indicated programming and recreation for these individuals.

Background to the Position Statement

The number of persons incarcerated in prisons and jails in the United States has risen dramatically during the past three decades, accompanied by a significant increase in prisoners with serious mental illness. Studies have consistently indicated that 8% to 19% of prison inmates have psychiatric disorders that result in significant functional disabilities and another 15% to 20% require some form of psychiatric intervention during their incarceration (Metzner 1993; Morrissey et al. 1993).

Physicians who work in U.S. correctional facilities face challenging working conditions, dual loyalties to patients and employers, and a tension between reasonable medical practices and the prison rules and culture. In recent years, physicians have increasingly confronted a new challenge: the prolonged solitary confinement, or segregation, of prisoners with serious mental illness. This prevalent corrections practice and the difficulties in providing access to care in these settings have received scant professional or academic attention (Metzner and Fellner 2010).

Segregated inmates are isolated from the general correctional population and receive services and activities apart from other inmates. For the purposes of this position statement, segregation refers to conditions of confinement characterized by an incarcerated person generally being locked in their cell for 23 hours or more per day (American Psychiatric Association 2000). Inmates may be segregated for institutional safety reasons (administrative segregation), disciplinary reasons (disciplinary segregation), or personal safety (protective custody) (National Commission on Correctional Health 2008). Correctional systems vary regarding the specific conditions of confinement in segregation units (e.g., one to two inmates in a cell, inmate access to a radio or television, other property restrictions, visitation privileges, etc.). The definition of "prolonged segregation" will, in part, depend on the conditions of confinement. In general, prolonged segregation means duration of greater than 3–4 weeks.

Several studies have shown that inmates with serious mental illness have more difficulty adapting to prison life than do inmates without a serious mental illness. Morgan et al. (1993) reported that seriously mentally ill prisoners were less able to successfully negotiate the complexity of the prison environment, resulting in an increased number of rule infractions leading to more time in segregation and in prison. Lovell and Jemelka (1996, 1998) found that inmates with serious mental illnesses committed infractions at three times the rate of non-seriously mentally ill counterparts.

Placement of inmates with a serious mental illness in these settings can be contraindicated because of the potential for the psychiatric conditions to clinically deteriorate or not improve (American Psychiatric Association 1997; Metzner and Dvoskin 2006). Inmates with a serious mental illness who are a high suicide risk or demonstrating active psychotic symptoms should not be placed in segregation housing as previously defined and instead should be transferred to an acute psychiatric setting for stabilization.

References

American Psychiatric Association: Practice guideline for the treatment of patients with schizophrenia. Am J Psychiatry 154(4 suppl):1–63, 1997 9090368

American Psychiatric Association: Psychiatric Services in Jails and Prisons, 2nd Edition. Washington, DC, American Psychiatric Association, 2000

Lovell D, Jemelka R: When inmates misbehave: the costs of discipline. The Prison Journal 76:165–179, 1996

Lovell D, Jemelka R: Coping with mental illness in prison. Family and Community Health 21:54–66, 1998

Metzner JL: Guidelines for psychiatric services in prisons. Crim Behav Ment Health 3:252–267, 1993

Metzner JL, Dvoskin JA: An overview of correctional psychiatry. Psychiatr Clin North Am 29:761–772, 2006 16904510

Metzner JL, Fellner J: Solitary confinement and mental illness in U.S. prisons: a challenge for medical ethics. J Am Acad Psychiatry Law 38:104–108, 2010 20305083

Morgan DW, Edwards AC, Faulkner LR: The adaptation to prison by individuals with schizophrenia. Bull Am Acad Psychiatry Law 21:427–433, 1993 8054673

Morrissey JP, Swanson JW, Goldstrom I, et al: Overview of Mental Health Services by State Adult Correctional Facilities: United States, 1988 (DHHS Publ No SMA 93-1993). Washington, DC, U.S. Department of Health and Human Services, 1993, pp 1–13

National Commission on Correctional Health: Standards for Mental Health Services in Correctional Facilities. Chicago, IL, National Commission on Correctional Health, 2008

Index

*Page numbers printed in **boldface** type refer to tables or figures.*